CORE STRENGTH AND FLEXIBILITY THROUGH PILATES:

Transform Your Body with Targeted Exercises.

SMITH WALKER

DEDICATION

To my family, whose unwavering support and love have been my foundation,

To my friends, who have inspired and encouraged me every step of the way,

And to all the dreamers and doers, who strive for success and never give up,

This book is dedicated to you.

May it be a guide and a source of inspiration on your journey to achieving your dreams.

With heartfelt gratitude.

TABLE OF CONTENT

Introduction: The Power of Pilates for Core Strength and Flexibility

Pilates is much more than just a fitness trend; it's a comprehensive mind-body discipline that strengthens, stretches, and aligns the body while cultivating mindfulness and balance. Whether you're new to Pilates or looking to deepen your understanding of its transformative potential, this introduction explores how Pilates fosters core strength, flexibility, and overall well-being. Through a combination of history, core-focused insights, and an overview of how this book will guide you, you'll discover how Pilates can transform both your body and mind.

What is Pilates? The History and Philosophy of Pilates as a Mind-Body Discipline

Pilates was developed in the early 20th century by Joseph Pilates, a physical trainer who believed in the connection between the mind and body to achieve optimal health. Originally termed "Contrology," Pilates' method was designed to help people improve their physical capabilities by focusing on controlled, precise movements, breathing techniques, and mental focus. It was first popularized by dancers and athletes, but it has since evolved into a widely practiced form of exercise across all fitness levels.

The core philosophy of Pilates centers around six key principles: concentration, control, centering, flow, precision, and breath. Each of these principles emphasizes the importance of aligning the body and mind to create a harmonious and balanced approach to fitness. Pilates focuses on stabilizing the core—often referred to as the "powerhouse" of the body—before initiating movement from other parts of the body. This mindful movement supports the development of strength, flexibility, and overall physical health while fostering mental clarity and stress reduction.

In this book, you'll learn not just the movements of Pilates but how to apply its principles in a way that maximizes their impact on your core strength and flexibility.

The Importance of Core Strength: How a Strong Core Supports Overall Health, Posture, and Movement

Core strength is foundational to almost every movement we make. Whether you're bending down to pick something up, walking, running, or lifting weights, your core plays a crucial role in stabilizing your spine and pelvis, protecting you from injury, and improving your balance and posture.

The core consists of the abdominal muscles, lower back, obliques, pelvic floor, diaphragm, and even the muscles around the hips. These muscles work together to create a stable base for movement and play a significant role in maintaining proper posture. Poor core strength can lead to a variety of issues, such as lower back pain, poor posture, and an increased risk of injury during physical activities.

Pilates is unique in that it places the core at the center of every exercise. The controlled, deliberate movements of Pilates engage your deep core muscles, helping to build strength from the inside out. As you work through the Pilates exercises outlined in this book, you'll notice improvements not only in your core strength but also in your ability to move through daily life with more stability and ease.

The Role of Flexibility: How Flexibility Complements Strength, Aids in Injury Prevention, and Enhances Functional Movement

Flexibility is often undervalued in traditional strength training, but in Pilates, flexibility is just as important as core strength. Flexibility allows for full, unimpeded range of motion in the muscles and joints, which not only helps prevent injury but also improves overall functional movement. When muscles are tight or stiff, they can limit your movement, create imbalances in your body, and increase your risk of strains or sprains.

Pilates is known for its ability to lengthen and stretch the muscles as you build strength. Unlike static stretching or traditional flexibility training, Pilates uses dynamic, flowing movements to stretch the muscles in a controlled manner, enhancing their elasticity and pliability. As you progress through the exercises in this book, you'll develop a balanced mix of strength and flexibility, which will help you move more freely and comfortably in both your workouts and daily activities.

Pilates also emphasizes the connection between strength and flexibility—strong muscles need to be flexible to function optimally. In this book, you will learn how to improve flexibility through targeted exercises, ensuring that your body remains balanced and free from injury.

How Pilates Transforms Your Body: The Holistic Benefits of Pilates Beyond Physical Appearance—Mental Clarity, Balance, and Body Awareness

While Pilates certainly helps to tone and strengthen the body, its true power lies in its holistic benefits. Pilates goes beyond physical fitness to improve mental well-being, enhance body awareness, and promote balance in all areas of life.

One of the key aspects of Pilates is its focus on breath and mindfulness. Controlled breathing not only helps you engage your core and other muscles more effectively but also reduces stress and promotes relaxation. This mindful approach to movement fosters a deeper connection between the mind and body, which can lead to greater mental clarity and focus.

Pilates also improves balance and coordination, both physically and mentally. The emphasis on proper alignment and controlled movement forces you to be present in each exercise, which enhances your ability to focus and tune into your body's needs. This heightened sense of body awareness helps prevent injury and promotes better movement patterns, both during workouts and in daily life.

As you work through the targeted Pilates exercises in this book, you'll notice how Pilates not only transforms your body but also your mindset. You'll develop a stronger, more flexible body and a clearer, more focused mind.

Overview of the Book: How This Guide Will Help You Develop Core Strength and Flexibility Through Targeted Pilates Exercises

This book is designed to guide you on a journey of physical and mental transformation through Pilates. Whether your goal is to build core strength, increase flexibility, or simply improve your overall well-being, this book offers practical exercises, routines, and insights to help you achieve your goals.

Throughout the chapters, you will find:

- Detailed explanations of core-focused Pilates exercises, with clear instructions on how to perform them safely and effectively.
- Flexibility-enhancing exercises that will lengthen and stretch your muscles, improving your range of motion and reducing the risk of injury.
- Tips on how to incorporate Pilates into your daily life to maximize its benefits.
- Suggestions for progressing your practice as you get stronger and more flexible, ensuring that your Pilates journey continues to evolve.

Whether you're a beginner or a seasoned practitioner, this book offers something for everyone. By the end of this guide, you'll not only have a stronger core and more flexible body but also a deeper understanding of how to maintain and build upon these benefits for long-term health and wellness.

Part 1: Foundations of Core Strength and Flexibility

Chapter 1: Understanding Core Anatomy and Function

The core serves as the powerhouse of the body, crucial for stabilizing, supporting, and controlling movement. In this chapter, we'll take a closer look at the muscles that make up the core, how they function in everyday activities, and why Pilates is uniquely suited to developing core strength.

The Core Muscles: A Deep Dive into the Muscles That Make Up Your Core

The term "core" often conjures up thoughts of the abdominal muscles, but in reality, the core is a much larger and more complex system. It consists of several interconnected muscle groups, each playing a critical role in supporting the spine, pelvis, and overall body movement.

1. **Rectus Abdominis**
   This is the muscle most people think of when they hear "core." Commonly referred to as the "six-pack" muscle, the rectus abdominis runs vertically along the front of the abdomen. It's responsible for flexing the spine, which helps in movements like crunches or bending forward. However, its role in overall core strength is just one piece of the puzzle.

2. **Transverse Abdominis (TVA)**
   This muscle lies deep beneath the rectus abdominis and wraps around the torso like a corset. The TVA plays a critical role in stabilizing the spine and pelvis, especially during movement. It's engaged during almost every Pilates exercise, helping to create a strong, stable core that supports both movement and posture.

3. **Obliques (Internal and External)**
   The obliques run along the sides of the abdomen, with the external obliques sitting just beneath the skin and the internal obliques lying deeper. These muscles are responsible for lateral flexion (side bending), rotation of the torso, and supporting spinal stability. They are engaged in twisting movements, such as in Pilates exercises like the "Criss-Cross," where rotation and abdominal engagement are crucial.

4. **Pelvic Floor Muscles**
   Located at the base of the core, these muscles support the pelvic organs and help maintain bladder and bowel control. The pelvic floor is often overlooked in traditional workouts, but it plays a significant role in core stability and strength. In Pilates, activating the pelvic floor muscles helps stabilize the pelvis and lower back, ensuring safer and more effective movement.

5. **Diaphragm**
   The diaphragm is a large, dome-shaped muscle located beneath the lungs that plays a central role in breathing. In Pilates, breath control is

critical, and learning to engage the diaphragm properly supports better core engagement. When you breathe deeply and correctly, the diaphragm works with the pelvic floor and other core muscles to stabilize the trunk and create a foundation for movement.

6. **Erector Spinae**

   These muscles run along the spine and are responsible for extending the back. Strong erector spinae muscles are essential for maintaining an upright posture, especially when performing movements that require spinal extension. Pilates focuses on strengthening these muscles through exercises like the "Swan Dive," which involves controlled back extension to promote a balanced, flexible core.

7. **Multifidus**

   This deep spinal muscle stabilizes individual vertebrae during movement. It works in concert with the transverse abdominis and pelvic floor to provide stability to the spine, particularly during exercises that challenge balance and control.

By targeting all these muscles, Pilates creates a comprehensive approach to core strength. A balanced, strong core is not just about looking toned—it's about ensuring that every part of your body is supported and protected during movement.

Core Function in Everyday Movement

The core is engaged in almost every movement we make, from the simplest tasks like sitting up in bed or walking to more complex movements like lifting, jumping, or twisting. A weak core can lead to poor posture, lower back pain, and an increased risk of injury, while a strong core provides stability, control, and balance.

1. **Posture and Alignment**
   Core strength is fundamental to maintaining good posture. The muscles of the core hold the spine and pelvis in proper alignment, which is especially important when sitting or standing for extended periods. Weak core muscles can lead to slouching, which strains the lower back and shoulders, potentially causing chronic pain. Pilates focuses on training the deep core muscles to support a neutral spine, helping you maintain better posture throughout the day.

   Example: Imagine sitting at your desk for hours, hunched over your computer. Without strong core muscles to support your spine, this position can cause tension in the lower back and shoulders. But with a strong core, you can maintain an upright posture, reducing the risk of discomfort or injury.

2. **Everyday Activities**
   Many everyday tasks, like bending to pick something up, twisting to grab an object, or standing up from a chair, engage the core. The stronger your core, the more stable and

controlled these movements become. For example, lifting heavy objects without proper core engagement can lead to back injuries, but with core strength, your body is more equipped to handle the load safely.

Example: When you carry groceries, a strong core helps distribute the weight evenly, preventing strain on the lower back. In Pilates, exercises like the "Plank" and "Side Bend" help reinforce the core's role in stabilizing the body during such movements.

3. **Athletic Performance**
   Whether you're running, swimming, or playing a sport, core strength is essential. It improves balance, agility, and coordination, helping athletes perform more efficiently and with less risk of injury. A weak core can lead to compensations in other parts of the body, increasing the likelihood of strains and injuries.

   Example: A runner with a weak core may experience lower back pain due to poor posture and lack of stability. However, by engaging in Pilates exercises that target the core, such as "Hundreds" or "Leg Circles," they can strengthen their core muscles and improve their running form.

Pilates and the Core: Why Pilates is Particularly Effective for Core Strengthening

Pilates stands out as one of the most effective methods for core strengthening due to its emphasis on controlled movements and deep muscle engagement. Unlike traditional core exercises, such as crunches, which tend to focus primarily on the rectus abdominis, Pilates works all layers of the core, including the deep stabilizing muscles.

1. **Controlled Movements**
   Pilates emphasizes slow, controlled movements that require focus and precision. This allows for deeper engagement of the core muscles, particularly the transverse abdominis and pelvic floor. Each exercise is designed to activate these muscles, promoting stability and strength from the inside out.

   Example: In the "Pilates Roll-Up," you slowly engage each vertebra as you curl up and down, which activates the entire core, from the abdominals to the lower back. This is far more effective for developing functional core strength than fast, repetitive crunches.

2. **Breath   Control**
   Pilates integrates breath with movement, teaching practitioners how to engage their diaphragm and core muscles simultaneously. This breath control supports proper muscle activation and helps deepen the engagement of the core muscles.

Example: The "Hundreds" exercise involves coordinated breath patterns while maintaining core engagement. By breathing deeply into the ribcage, the diaphragm works in harmony with the abdominal muscles to strengthen and stabilize the core.

3. **Balanced Muscle Development**
Pilates ensures that all aspects of the core are worked evenly, promoting balance in the body. Many traditional exercises focus heavily on the front of the core, neglecting the muscles of the back and sides. Pilates, however, incorporates exercises that work the entire torso, ensuring balanced strength and stability.

Example: Exercises like "Side Planks" engage the obliques, while "Swan Dive" targets the muscles of the lower back, ensuring that both the front and back of the core are strengthened equally.

4. **Functional Strength**
Pilates exercises are designed to enhance functional movement, which means that the strength you develop in Pilates can be applied to everyday activities. By improving core strength through functional movement patterns, Pilates ensures that your body is better equipped to handle the demands of daily life.

Example: The "Bridge" exercise not only strengthens the core but also engages the glutes and hamstrings, muscles that are vital for movements like standing up, walking, or climbing stairs.

Through a deep understanding of core anatomy, its function in everyday life, and the unique benefits Pilates offers, you'll gain the knowledge and tools to build a strong, stable, and flexible core. This chapter lays the foundation for your journey, helping you appreciate the critical role your core plays in every movement, whether you're in the Pilates studio, at work, or out in the world.

Chapter 2: Flexibility and Its Importance

Flexibility plays a vital role in how we move and function in everyday life, enhancing mobility and helping to prevent injury. This chapter explores the concept of flexibility, the muscles involved, and how Pilates is designed to improve flexibility by stretching and lengthening muscles. By the end of this chapter, you'll understand why flexibility is a cornerstone of overall health and well-being and how Pilates can help you achieve a balanced, flexible body.

What is Flexibility?: Understanding Flexibility and Its Role in Functional Movement

Flexibility is the ability of muscles and joints to move through their full range of motion without discomfort or restriction. It's essential not just for athletes or dancers, but for anyone who wants to move with ease in daily life. Whether you're reaching for an object on a high shelf, bending down to tie your shoes, or turning to check your blind spot while driving, flexibility is crucial for maintaining functional, pain-free movement.

Functional Movement and Flexibility Functional movement refers to the body's ability to move in everyday life efficiently and without restriction. Flexibility is key to functional movement because it allows muscles and joints to move freely, reducing the risk of strains and imbalances. A lack of flexibility can lead to tightness, poor posture, and compensatory movements, which in turn can cause injury.

Example: Imagine reaching down to pick up something off the floor. Without flexibility in your hamstrings and lower back, this simple task could cause strain, leading to discomfort or even injury. Pilates enhances flexibility by promoting controlled, dynamic stretches that target key areas of tightness and improve range of motion.

Importance of Flexibility in Daily Activities Beyond just preventing injury, flexibility plays a major role in the ease and fluidity of movement. Tight, inflexible muscles can limit your ability to perform everyday tasks comfortably, from bending down to lift objects to stretching in ways that promote full mobility.

Example: Consider how flexibility impacts your ability to rotate your torso while gardening or twist around when backing up your car. In Pilates, exercises like "Spine Twist" and "Saw" help improve rotational flexibility, making such movements easier and safer.

Muscles Involved in Flexibility: Key Muscle Groups that Need Flexibility for Mobility and Injury Prevention

Certain muscle groups are particularly important when it comes to flexibility because they directly affect mobility and alignment. Tightness in these areas can limit movement and cause discomfort. In this section, we will explore some of the major muscle groups involved in flexibility and why their flexibility is crucial for mobility and injury prevention.

1. **Hamstrings**
   The hamstrings are a group of three muscles located at the back of your thighs. Tight hamstrings are a common issue, particularly for people who sit for long periods. Tightness in the hamstrings can lead to lower back pain, poor posture, and limited range of motion in the hips and legs.

   Example: Pilates exercises like the "Leg Circles" or the "Roll Over" target the hamstrings, helping to lengthen and release tension in these muscles. Over time, consistent stretching in Pilates helps improve flexibility in the hamstrings, which aids in more fluid leg movements.

2. **Hip Flexors**
   The hip flexors are a group of muscles located in the front of your hips that are responsible for lifting your knees and bending at the waist. Tight hip flexors can lead to lower back pain and restricted movement in the pelvis and legs. This is especially common in people who spend a lot of time sitting, as the hip flexors remain shortened during seated positions.

   Example: Pilates exercises like the "Lunge Stretch" or "Bridge" help to stretch and strengthen the hip flexors. By lengthening these muscles, Pilates can improve flexibility and reduce strain on the lower back, improving mobility and posture.

3. **Lower Back**
   The muscles in your lower back play a crucial role in supporting the spine and allowing for flexibility in bending and twisting movements. Tightness in the lower back can lead to discomfort and restrict movement in everyday activities.

   Example: The "Spine Stretch Forward" in Pilates is a classic exercise that helps release tension in the lower back, promoting flexibility and ease of movement through the spine. This exercise encourages lengthening and articulation of each vertebra, helping to alleviate stiffness and improve spinal mobility.

4. **Shoulders and Upper Back**
   The muscles around the shoulders and upper back are critical for arm and shoulder mobility. Tightness in these muscles can lead to poor posture, restricted arm movement, and discomfort in the neck and shoulders.

   Example: Pilates exercises like the "Arm Circles" and "Shoulder Bridge" focus on increasing the range of motion in the shoulders and upper back. These exercises help loosen tight muscles, making it easier to reach overhead, extend the arms, or perform tasks that require upper body flexibility.

How Pilates Enhances Flexibility: How Pilates Stretches and Lengthens Muscles for a Balanced, Flexible Body

One of the key principles of Pilates is elongation and flexibility of the muscles. Unlike other forms of exercise that focus primarily on strengthening muscles, Pilates incorporates dynamic stretching and controlled movement to lengthen and release tension. This approach not only enhances flexibility but also helps improve overall balance, posture, and functional movement.

1. **Dynamic Stretching in Pilates**
   Pilates combines strength with flexibility, which means that the exercises not only engage and strengthen muscles but also stretch them. By moving through full ranges of motion in a controlled manner, Pilates encourages the lengthening of muscles and the opening of joints.

   Example: The "Mermaid Stretch" is a Pilates exercise that lengthens the muscles on the sides of the body, including the obliques and intercostal muscles. As you reach and bend to the side, the muscles are dynamically stretched, improving both flexibility and spinal mobility.

2. **Active Stretching and Strengthening**
   In Pilates, flexibility is often developed through

active stretching, where muscles are lengthened while simultaneously engaging their opposing muscle groups. This active engagement enhances both strength and flexibility, promoting a balanced and controlled range of motion.

Example: In the "Single Leg Stretch," you alternate pulling one leg toward your chest while extending the other leg outward. This exercise not only strengthens the abdominals but also stretches the hamstrings and hip flexors, making it an effective way to build both flexibility and stability in the lower body.

3. **Joint Mobility and Flexibility** Pilates exercises are designed to enhance joint mobility by encouraging movements that rotate, stretch, and open the joints. This is particularly important for maintaining flexibility as we age because joints can become stiff and less mobile over time.

Example: The "Spinal Twist" exercise focuses on rotating the spine, promoting flexibility in the thoracic region of the back. This rotation helps release tightness in the upper back and shoulders while improving overall spinal mobility.

4. **Mind-Body Connection in Flexibility** Pilates emphasizes the importance of the mind-body connection. When practicing Pilates, you

are encouraged to be fully aware of your body's movements, paying attention to how your muscles stretch and contract. This awareness helps you engage the muscles more effectively, leading to deeper stretches and greater flexibility.

Example: During the "Roll Up," you are instructed to slowly articulate each vertebra of your spine as you curl up and down. This exercise requires concentration and control, allowing you to engage the deep core muscles while simultaneously stretching the spine and hamstrings.

Flexibility is not just about being able to stretch your muscles—it's about moving freely and comfortably in your daily life. Through the mindful practice of Pilates, you can develop both flexibility and strength, leading to better posture, reduced risk of injury, and more fluid movement. Whether you're new to Pilates or looking to deepen your practice, understanding how Pilates enhances flexibility will empower you to move with grace and ease.

Chapter 3: Pilates Principles for Strength and Flexibility

The essence of Pilates lies in its foundational principles, which guide every movement and posture to ensure proper alignment, control, and engagement of muscles. This chapter delves into the six key Pilates principles—Concentration, Control, Centering, Flow, Precision, and Breathing—explaining how they apply to building core strength and enhancing flexibility. Understanding and applying these principles will enable you to get the most out of your Pilates practice, maximizing both strength and flexibility.

The Six Pilates Principles: Concentration, Control, Centering, Flow, Precision, and Breathing

Joseph Pilates, the founder of the Pilates method, developed six guiding principles that form the backbone of the practice. These principles are designed to help you cultivate mind-body awareness and execute movements with intention and precision. Let's break down each principle and its significance for both strength and flexibility.

1. **Concentration**
   Pilates is a mind-body discipline, and concentration is at the heart of this connection. Every movement in Pilates requires full mental focus to ensure you're engaging the right muscles and maintaining proper form. This focus allows you to control your body more

effectively, making each movement purposeful and beneficial.

Example: While performing the "Hundred," concentrating on maintaining your abdominal engagement and keeping your lower back grounded is essential. Without focus, the exercise may lose its effectiveness, but with concentration, it builds core strength by ensuring that you are using the proper muscles to stabilize the torso.

2. **Control**
   In Pilates, control is key to preventing injury and ensuring that you are moving with intention rather than momentum. Each movement, no matter how small or large, should be controlled, using the core to stabilize the body. Control prevents sloppy movements and enhances the overall effectiveness of the exercises.

   Example: In the "Leg Circles" exercise, it's tempting to let the momentum of your leg carry the movement. However, by controlling the movement from the core, you engage your stabilizing muscles, improving both core strength and hip flexibility.

3. **Centering**
   The core, often referred to as the "powerhouse" in Pilates, is the center of all movement. By focusing on centering your body, you activate the muscles of your abdominals, lower back,

and pelvic floor. This principle ensures that all movements originate from the core, leading to better stability, balance, and strength.

Example: In the "Plank" exercise, centering ensures that you are using your core to support the body, rather than relying on your arms or shoulders. This not only builds core strength but also improves overall alignment and posture.

4. **Flow**
   Pilates emphasizes smooth, continuous movement, rather than jerky or disjointed motions. Flow refers to the graceful transition from one movement to the next, creating a sense of rhythm and fluidity. By moving with flow, you not only enhance flexibility but also promote better circulation and mobility.

   Example: The "Swan Dive" is a great example of flow in Pilates. The exercise involves arching the back in a controlled manner and then smoothly transitioning into the dive, which promotes spinal flexibility and strengthens the back muscles.

5. **Precision**
   Pilates is about quality, not quantity. Precision ensures that each movement is executed with exactness, engaging the proper muscles and avoiding compensatory movements. When movements are precise, you maximize their benefits while minimizing the risk of injury.

Example: The "Roll-Up" is a perfect demonstration of precision. This exercise requires exact control of each vertebra as you slowly peel your spine off the mat and then roll back down. By focusing on precision, you ensure that you are engaging your core and stretching your spine correctly.

6. **Breathing**
   Breathing in Pilates is not just about oxygenating the body—it's about creating a rhythm that supports movement and engages the core. Inhaling helps you prepare for movement, while exhaling aids in deepening the engagement of your core muscles. Proper breathing also helps release tension and promotes relaxation, making stretching more effective.

   Example: In the "Spine Stretch Forward" exercise, inhaling allows you to prepare for the movement, while exhaling helps you deepen the stretch as you reach forward, releasing tension in the spine and improving flexibility.

How These Principles Apply to Core Strength: Practical Tips on Focusing on the Core with Proper Form

Each Pilates principle plays a unique role in strengthening the core. By understanding and applying these principles, you can optimize your workout to focus on core stability and strength. Let's explore how these principles contribute to core development:

1. **Concentration and Core Engagement**
   Core strength requires focused engagement of the deep stabilizing muscles, such as the transverse abdominis and pelvic floor. Concentrating on drawing your navel toward your spine during exercises ensures that you're activating these muscles effectively.

   Tip: In exercises like the "Double Leg Stretch," focus on keeping your lower back grounded and engaging your abdominals as you extend your legs. This concentration prevents your back from arching and ensures that the core is doing the work.

2. **Control and Core Stability**
   Core exercises are most effective when performed with controlled movements, ensuring that you're not relying on momentum. Slower, more deliberate movements allow you to feel the deep engagement of the core muscles.

   Tip: While performing "Side Planks," move slowly into the plank position, engaging your obliques and transverse abdominis for stability. The control prevents your hips from sagging and ensures maximum core engagement.

3. **Centering and Core Activation**
   Centering ensures that your movements are initiated from your core, rather than relying on

the extremities. This concept is central to Pilates and is essential for developing core strength.

Tip: In the "Teaser," focus on lifting your torso from your core, not your arms or legs. This focus on centering allows for a stronger, more stable movement that builds core strength effectively.

Applying These Principles to Flexibility: How to Stretch Safely and Effectively by Using These Foundational Principles

Just as these principles apply to strengthening the core, they are equally important in enhancing flexibility. Flexibility in Pilates is achieved through controlled, precise movements that safely stretch and lengthen the muscles. Here's how you can apply the principles to your flexibility training:

1. **Concentration and Flexibility**
   Concentration helps you tune into your body's sensations during a stretch, allowing you to find your edge without overstretching. By concentrating on your breath and the feeling of the stretch, you can deepen your flexibility safely.

   Tip: During the "Hamstring Stretch," focus on maintaining an even stretch through the back of your leg. Concentrating on how your body feels helps prevent overstretching, which could lead to injury.

2. **Control and Stretching Safely**
   Controlled stretching in Pilates ensures that you are lengthening the muscles safely without bouncing or jerking into a stretch. This gradual approach reduces the risk of muscle strain.

   Tip: In the "Saw" exercise, control the rotation of your spine as you reach forward, ensuring that the movement is slow and deliberate. This controlled motion helps stretch the hamstrings and back muscles without overstretching.

3. **Flow and Flexibility**
   Flow is crucial in stretching, as it helps to gently increase range of motion over time. Flowing through stretches with smooth, continuous movements prevents muscle tension from building up.

   Tip: In the "Mermaid Stretch," focus on flowing from one side to the other, creating a fluid motion that opens up the side body and improves flexibility in the obliques and intercostal muscles.

4. **Precision and Effective Stretching**
   Precision in stretching ensures that you are targeting the correct muscles. Proper alignment during stretches helps you get the most benefit while avoiding compensatory movements that can reduce the effectiveness of the stretch.

   Tip: In the "Spine Stretch Forward," make sure your shoulders stay down and your back remains straight as you reach forward. This precise alignment ensures that you are effectively stretching the spine and hamstrings.

By applying the Pilates principles of concentration, control, centering, flow, precision, and breathing, you can safely and effectively enhance both core strength and flexibility. These principles guide your movements, ensuring that you stretch and strengthen with purpose, mindfulness, and alignment. As you continue your Pilates journey, these foundational concepts will support your progress, helping you to move with greater ease, strength, and fluidity.

Part 2: Core-Focused Pilates Exercises

Chapter 4: Beginner Pilates Core Exercises

Pilates is renowned for its ability to build a strong, stable core, often referred to as the "powerhouse" of the body. The core muscles extend beyond just the visible six-pack abs; they encompass the deep abdominal muscles, pelvic floor, diaphragm, and the muscles around the lower back. In this chapter, we will explore beginner-level Pilates exercises that focus on engaging the deep core muscles to lay a solid foundation for strength, stability, and improved posture. Additionally, we will discuss the role of proper breathing in core activation and how to integrate diaphragmatic breathing into your Pilates practice.

Engaging the Deep Core Muscles: Exercises that Help You Connect with Your Deep Core Muscles

One of the main goals of Pilates is to target the deep core muscles, which are essential for supporting your spine, improving balance, and providing the stability needed for everyday movements. The exercises outlined below are perfect for beginners as they emphasize slow, controlled movements, making it easier to connect with the deep core.

The Hundred

The Hundred is one of the most iconic Pilates exercises and an excellent way to warm up the body while engaging the core. This exercise challenges the abdominal muscles and improves circulation through rhythmic breathing.

1. **How to Perform:**
   - Lie flat on your back with your legs lifted to tabletop position (knees bent at a 90-degree angle).
   - Lift your head, neck, and shoulders off the mat, reaching your arms forward so they are parallel to the floor.
   - Begin to pump your arms up and down in small, controlled movements.
   - Inhale for five arm pumps, then exhale for five arm pumps. Repeat until you reach 100 pumps (hence the name).
   - Keep your abdominals engaged and your lower back pressed into the mat throughout the exercise.
2. **Core Engagement Tips:**
   - Focus on pulling your navel toward your spine to engage the transverse abdominis, the deepest layer of your abdominal muscles.
   - If you feel strain in your neck, lower your head back onto the mat while keeping the rest of your body in position.
3. **Modifications:**
   - For a more accessible variation, keep your feet on the mat instead of lifting them into tabletop.

o As you build strength, extend your legs straight out at a 45-degree angle to increase the challenge for your core

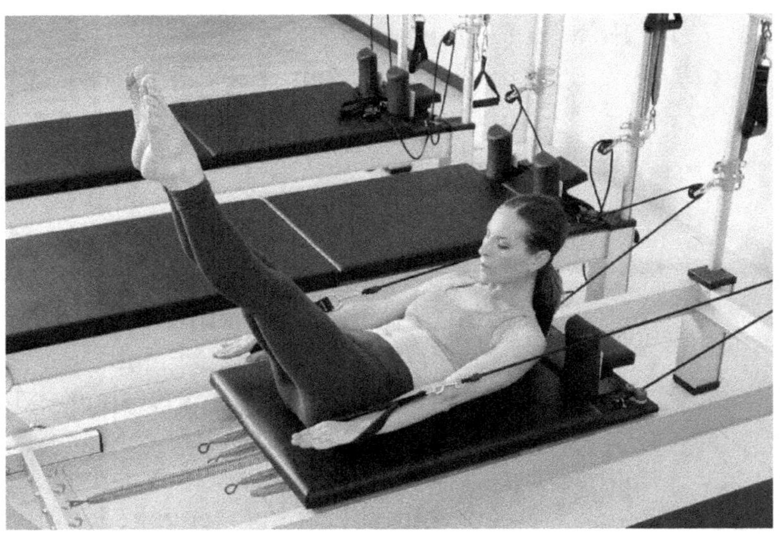

Single Leg Stretch

The **Single Leg Stretch** is a beginner-friendly exercise that isolates each side of the body while keeping the core engaged. It improves coordination and helps to strengthen both the deep and superficial abdominal muscles.

1. **How to Perform:**
   o Lie on your back with your legs in tabletop position.
   o Lift your head, neck, and shoulders off the mat, and bring your right knee toward your chest while extending your left leg out at a 45-degree angle.

- Hold your right knee with both hands and alternate legs, pulling the left knee in as you extend the right leg.
- Continue alternating for 10-12 repetitions on each side, maintaining your head lifted and your core engaged.

2. **Core Engagement Tips:**
   - Imagine your navel pulling down toward the mat, ensuring your lower back stays pressed into the floor.
   - Keep your movements controlled, focusing on engaging your core rather than relying on momentum to switch legs.

3. **Modifications:**
   - If you experience discomfort in your neck, rest your head on the mat while continuing the leg movements.
   - For a more challenging variation, extend your legs lower to the floor, but only if you can keep your lower back grounded.

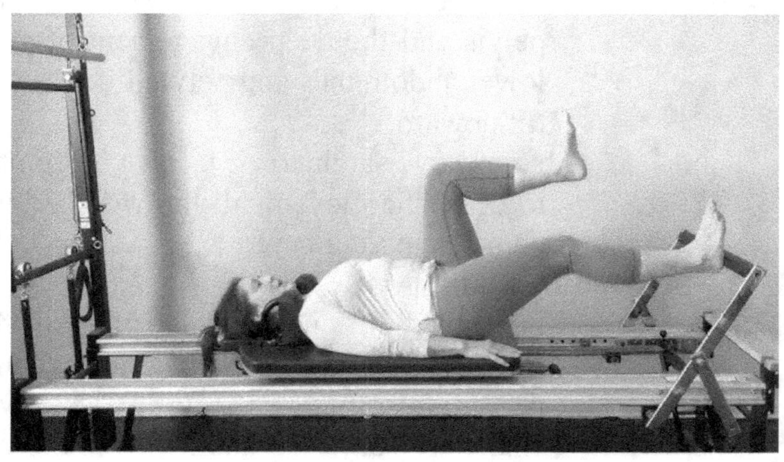

Pelvic Tilts

Pelvic Tilts are a simple yet highly effective exercise for connecting with the deep core and pelvic floor muscles. They are perfect for beginners as they focus on gentle core activation and improving lower back mobility.

1. **How to Perform:**
   - Lie on your back with your knees bent and feet flat on the floor, hip-width apart.
   - Place your hands on your hips to feel the movement of your pelvis.
   - On an exhale, gently tilt your pelvis upward, pressing your lower back into the mat and engaging your abdominals.
   - On an inhale, release the tilt, allowing a small curve to form in your lower back.
   - Repeat for 10-15 slow and controlled repetitions.
2. **Core Engagement Tips:**
   - Focus on the subtle movement of your pelvis and the deep engagement of your lower abdominals and pelvic floor as you tilt upward.
   - Avoid over-arching or using your glutes to drive the movement; the work should come from your core.
3. **Modifications:**
   - For added difficulty, lift your feet off the floor into tabletop position while performing the pelvic tilts. This will challenge your core stability even more.

Breathing for Core Activation: How to Use Diaphragmatic Breathing to Engage the Core Effectively

In Pilates, breathing plays a crucial role in both movement execution and core engagement. Diaphragmatic breathing, or belly breathing, helps to activate the core muscles, particularly the transverse abdominis, which acts as an internal corset around your midsection.

1. **Understanding Diaphragmatic Breathing:** Diaphragmatic breathing involves inhaling deeply through the nose, allowing the diaphragm to expand and the belly to rise, and then exhaling completely, drawing the belly inward and engaging the deep core muscles. This type of breathing enhances oxygen flow, relaxes the body, and increases core stability.
2. **How to Practice Diaphragmatic Breathing for Core Activation:**
   - Sit or lie down in a comfortable position.
   - Place one hand on your chest and the other on your abdomen.
   - Inhale deeply through your nose, allowing your belly to rise while keeping your chest still.
   - As you exhale, pull your navel in toward your spine, engaging your deep core muscles.
   - Practice this breathing pattern for several cycles, focusing on activating the core on each exhale.

3. **Incorporating Breathing into Pilates Exercises:**
   - In **The Hundred**, focus on exhaling as you pump your arms, engaging your core with each breath out.
   - In **Single Leg Stretch**, inhale as you pull one leg in, and exhale as you switch legs, using the breath to drive the movement and keep the core engaged.
   - In **Pelvic Tilts**, exhale as you tilt your pelvis upward, focusing on the engagement of your lower abdominals and pelvic floor.

Practical Example: Connecting Breath and Movement

Let's put it all together in a short, flowing sequence:

- Start in a **Supine Position** (lying on your back) with your knees bent and feet flat on the mat.
- Inhale deeply, letting your belly rise, and on the exhale, engage your core and perform a **Pelvic Tilt**, pressing your lower back into the mat.
- Transition into **The Hundred** by lifting your legs to tabletop and pumping your arms, using diaphragmatic breathing to maintain core activation.
- Move into **Single Leg Stretch** by alternating legs, continuing to breathe deeply and engage the core on each exhale.

This sequence highlights how breath and core engagement work hand in hand in Pilates, even in beginner-level exercises. By mastering these fundamental movements and breathing techniques, you'll lay a strong foundation for more advanced Pilates practice in the future.

Summary

By focusing on the deep core muscles, beginners can build a strong foundation of stability and strength. Exercises like **The Hundred**, **Single Leg Stretch**, and **Pelvic Tilts** introduce the basic movements and principles of Pilates while emphasizing the importance of core engagement. Additionally, diaphragmatic breathing plays a crucial role in core activation, supporting your practice by ensuring that each movement is mindful, controlled, and effective. These beginner exercises not only strengthen the core but also pave the way for more advanced Pilates work, offering lifelong benefits to posture, balance, and overall body strength.

Chapter 5: Intermediate Core Strengthening Exercises

Once you've built a solid foundation with beginner Pilates exercises, you're ready to progress to more challenging movements that increase core engagement and overall strength. Intermediate Pilates exercises take the basic principles of control, precision, and breath and introduce greater range of motion, deeper muscle activation, and new props to enhance your practice. This chapter focuses on strengthening the core through exercises like **The Roll-Up, Double Leg Stretch**, and **Plank Variations**, as well as how to incorporate Pilates props, such as the ring, ball, and band, to amplify the workout intensity.

Increasing Core Engagement and Challenge

As you move into intermediate Pilates, core engagement becomes even more crucial. The exercises in this section demand greater abdominal strength, control, and coordination. Let's dive into three highly effective intermediate exercises that will help you take your core strength to the next level.

The Roll-Up

The Roll-Up is a classic Pilates exercise that targets the entire core, particularly the rectus abdominis and obliques. It's a more challenging version of the basic **Pelvic Tilt** or **Crunch**, requiring you to lift your body off the mat with control.

1. **How to Perform:**
   - Begin lying on your back with your legs extended straight and arms reaching overhead.
   - Inhale as you bring your arms toward the ceiling, and slowly lift your head, neck, and shoulders off the mat.
   - Exhale as you continue to roll your spine up and forward, reaching toward your toes.
   - Inhale as you begin to roll back down, one vertebra at a time, using your core muscles to control the descent.
   - Repeat for 5-8 slow, controlled repetitions.
2. **Core Engagement Tips:**
   - Focus on initiating the movement from your deep core muscles (transverse abdominis) rather than using momentum.
   - If you struggle with the full movement, bend your knees slightly or use a Pilates strap around your feet for support.
3. **Benefits:**
   - **The Roll-Up** not only strengthens the core but also increases flexibility in the spine and hamstrings.
   - It challenges you to use both the front and back of your body to perform a controlled, fluid motion.

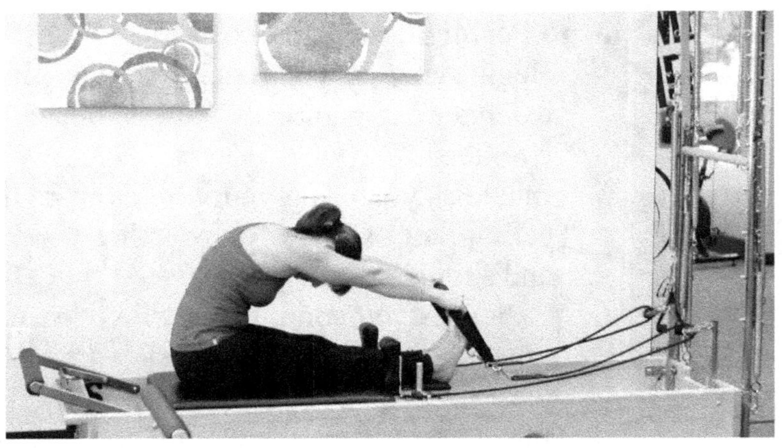

Double Leg Stretch

The **Double Leg Stretch** is another intermediate Pilates exercise that challenges both your core stability and your coordination. It works the entire abdominal region, particularly the deep core muscles that support the spine.

1. **How to Perform:**
    - Begin lying on your back with your legs in tabletop position and your arms reaching toward your shins.
    - Inhale as you extend both arms overhead and both legs straight out at a 45-degree angle.
    - Exhale as you sweep your arms back around and draw your knees toward your chest, returning to the starting position.
    - Repeat for 8-10 repetitions, maintaining control throughout.
2. **Core Engagement Tips:**

- o Be sure to keep your lower back pressed into the mat as you extend your legs to prevent strain or arching.
  - o Focus on breathing deeply and using the breath to initiate the movement, especially when pulling your knees back toward your chest.

3. **Modifications:**
   - o If extending both legs straight feels too challenging, you can perform the exercise with your knees bent or lower your legs only slightly.

4. **Benefits:**
   - o The **Double Leg Stretch** is excellent for building strength and endurance in the core, as well as improving coordination between the arms and legs.

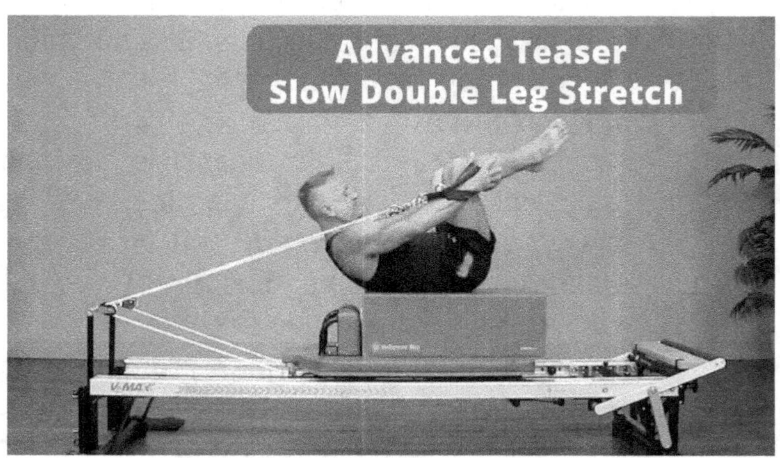

Plank Variations

Plank Variations are a more advanced way to engage the entire core, as well as the shoulders, arms, and legs. Planks target the deep stabilizing muscles of the core while also challenging your balance and endurance.

1. **How to Perform a Basic Plank:**
   - Start in a prone position (on your belly) and then lift yourself up onto your hands and toes, forming a straight line from head to heels.
   - Hold for 20-30 seconds, focusing on keeping your core tight, your back flat, and your shoulders stacked over your wrists.
   - As you advance, you can increase the duration of the plank or add variations like lifting one arm or leg.
2. **Plank Variations:**
   - **Side Plank:** From a plank position, rotate your body to one side, stacking your feet and extending one arm toward the ceiling. Hold for 20-30 seconds before switching sides.
   - **Plank with Leg Lift:** From a basic plank, lift one leg off the floor, hold for 5 seconds, then switch legs. This variation challenges your balance and adds extra core engagement.
   - **Forearm Plank:** This variation places you on your forearms instead of your

hands, which can reduce wrist strain while focusing more on the core and shoulders.

3. **Benefits:**
    o Planks are one of the most effective exercises for overall core strength, as they engage multiple muscle groups at once.
    o The added variations provide even more challenge to the stabilizing muscles of the core, hips, and shoulders.

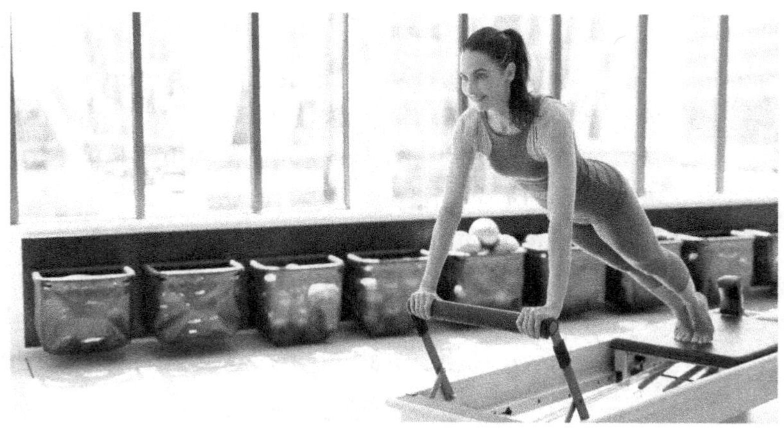

Using Props to Enhance Core Strength

Adding Pilates props, such as a ring, ball, or band, can intensify your core workout by increasing resistance and instability. These tools help to engage smaller stabilizing muscles and enhance the overall challenge of each exercise.

Pilates Ring

The **Pilates Ring** (or magic circle) is a small, flexible ring that provides resistance when squeezed. It can be used in a variety of exercises to engage the core and other muscle groups.

1. **Using the Ring for Core Engagement:**
   - In a **Seated Roll-Up**, place the ring between your hands and press inward as you roll up, engaging the core and chest simultaneously.
   - In a **Bridge** position, place the ring between your thighs and squeeze as you lift your hips. This adds an extra challenge to your inner thighs and lower abdominals.
2. **Core Benefits:**
   - The ring provides extra resistance, making core exercises more challenging while helping to tone the arms and legs as well.

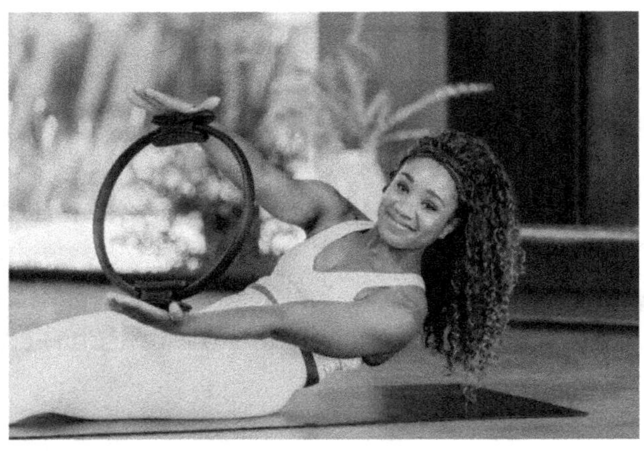

Pilates Ball

The **Pilates Ball** is a soft, inflatable ball that can be used to increase instability, which forces the core to work harder to stabilize the body during exercises.

1. **Using the Ball for Core Engagement:**
   - Place the ball under your lower back during **Crunches** to increase the range of motion and make the core muscles work harder.
   - In a **Plank**, place the ball under your shins to challenge your stability and balance, engaging the entire core.
2. **Core Benefits:**
   - The ball creates an unstable surface, forcing the core to work harder to maintain balance. This intensifies the workout and improves overall core strength.

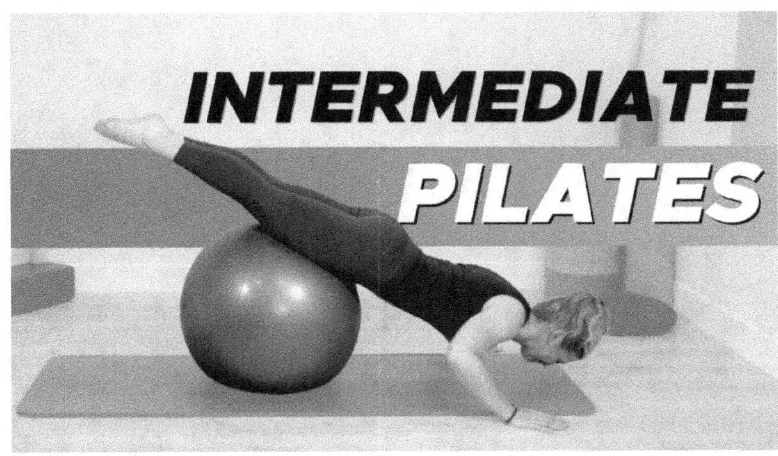

Resistance Bands

Resistance Bands are versatile tools that add resistance to any Pilates exercise, increasing the challenge for the core and other muscle groups.

1. **Using Bands for Core Engagement:**
   - In a **Double Leg Stretch**, loop the band around your feet and hold the ends in your hands. This adds resistance as you extend your legs, making the exercise more challenging for the core.
   - During **Planks**, place the band around your thighs and perform **Leg Lifts**. The added resistance increases glute and core engagement.
2. **Core Benefits:**
   - Bands provide constant tension, which helps to engage the core muscles more deeply and build strength through resistance training.

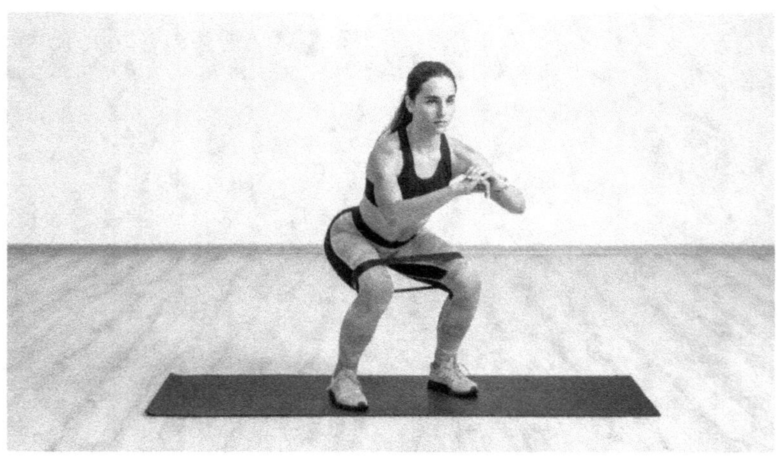

Summary

By progressing from beginner to intermediate Pilates exercises, you increase the challenge to your core muscles while enhancing strength, flexibility, and coordination. Exercises like **The Roll-Up**, **Double Leg Stretch**, and various **Plank Variations** introduce more complex movements that require greater core engagement. Adding Pilates props such as the ring, ball, and resistance bands further intensifies the workout, targeting stabilizing muscles and improving overall strength. With these intermediate exercises, you'll continue to build a strong, flexible, and resilient core, setting the stage for even more advanced Pilates practice in the future.

Chapter 6: Advanced Core Pilates Exercises

As you progress in your Pilates practice, advanced exercises offer an exciting challenge by engaging the entire body while focusing on deep core muscles. These advanced movements demand superior control, coordination, and strength, pushing your Pilates routine to a higher level. In this chapter, we will explore exercises like the **Teaser, Corkscrew**, and **Jackknife**, which test your balance and precision. Additionally, we'll introduce how to integrate the **Pilates Reformer** into your routine, enhancing core strength with machine-assisted exercises.

Challenging the Core with Full-Body Movements

Advanced Pilates exercises take core engagement to a whole new level by involving the entire body in complex, flowing motions. These exercises not only work the deep abdominal muscles but also challenge the arms, legs, and back. They require exceptional core stability and control, as well as flexibility and coordination.

Teaser

The **Teaser** is a signature Pilates exercise that combines abdominal strength, balance, and flexibility. It's one of the most challenging movements in Pilates and requires precise control to lift and balance the body.

1. **How to Perform:**

- o Start lying on your back with your arms extended overhead and legs straight.
- o Inhale as you raise your arms toward the ceiling, and simultaneously begin to lift your head, shoulders, and legs off the mat.
- o Exhale as you balance on your sitting bones, creating a V-shape with your body, with arms reaching forward toward your toes.
- o Hold for a few seconds, then inhale as you slowly roll back down with control, keeping your legs lifted until your back touches the mat.
- o Repeat for 3-5 repetitions.

2. **Core Engagement Tips:**
- o Focus on engaging your deep abdominal muscles (transverse abdominis) to control the movement, rather than using momentum.
- o Keep your back long and straight during the balancing phase, and avoid collapsing the chest.

3. **Modifications:**
- o If the full **Teaser** is too difficult, try performing the movement with bent knees or holding the position with one leg lifted at a time.

4. **Benefits:**
- o The **Teaser** strengthens the entire core, improves balance, and enhances flexibility in the hamstrings and spine. It

also promotes full-body coordination and control.

Teaser on the Reformer

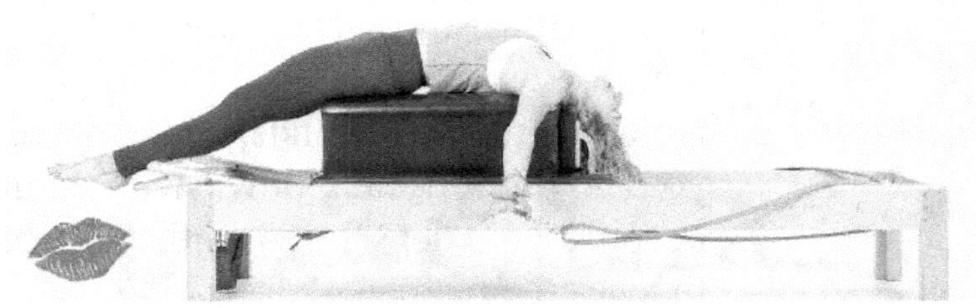

Corkscrew

The **Corkscrew** is an advanced Pilates exercise that works the obliques, lower abdominals, and hips. It also enhances spinal flexibility and control by involving a twisting motion.

1. **How to Perform:**
   - Begin lying on your back with your legs extended straight up toward the ceiling.
   - Inhale as you engage your core and lift your hips slightly off the mat, rolling your legs in a circular motion to the right, down, and to the left.
   - Exhale as you return to the starting position, using your core muscles to control the movement.

- o Repeat for 3-5 repetitions in each direction, alternating sides.
2. **Core Engagement Tips:**
   - o Keep your core muscles tight and control the movement throughout the exercise to avoid swinging or using momentum.
   - o Ensure your shoulders remain grounded on the mat as your legs circle, isolating the movement in your core and lower body.
3. **Modifications:**
   - o If lifting your hips off the mat is too challenging, perform the circular motion with your hips grounded, focusing on engaging your obliques.
4. **Benefits:**
   - o The **Corkscrew** targets the obliques and lower abdominals while promoting spinal mobility and control. It also helps to improve coordination between the upper and lower body.

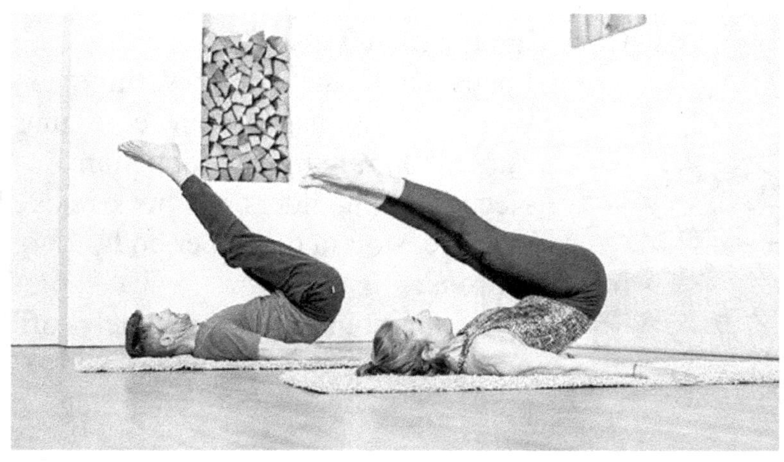

Jackknife

The **Jackknife** is a powerful core exercise that engages the entire abdominal region, with a focus on the lower abs and hip flexors. It requires a combination of strength, flexibility, and control to lift and lower the body in a controlled manner.

1. **How to Perform:**
    - Lie on your back with your arms by your sides, palms facing down.
    - Inhale as you lift your legs straight toward the ceiling, then continue lifting your hips and lower back off the mat until your legs are parallel to the floor behind your head (similar to a **Shoulder Stand**).
    - Exhale as you slowly lower your hips back down, maintaining control as you lower your legs toward the floor, stopping just above the mat.
    - Repeat for 5-8 repetitions.
2. **Core Engagement Tips:**
    - Focus on lifting and lowering the legs with control, using your core muscles rather than relying on momentum.
    - Keep your shoulders and neck relaxed to avoid tension in the upper body.
3. **Modifications:**
    - If lifting your hips completely off the mat is too challenging, practice the movement by lifting your legs only

partway, focusing on controlling the
descent.

4. **Benefits:**
   - The **Jackknife** strengthens the lower
     abdominals, improves spinal flexibility,
     and enhances balance and coordination.
     It also challenges the stabilizing muscles
     in the back and shoulders.

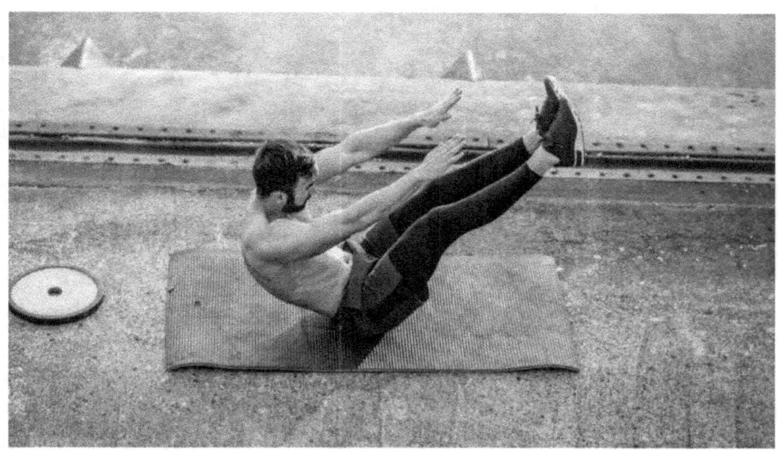

Using the Reformer for Core Strength

The **Pilates Reformer** is a versatile piece of
equipment that can significantly enhance core strength
by adding resistance, support, and variety to your
workout. It allows you to perform advanced exercises
with greater precision and control, making it ideal for
targeting deep core muscles.

Introduction to the Pilates Reformer

The **Reformer** consists of a flat platform, called a carriage, which moves along tracks. Resistance is provided by springs attached to the carriage, and exercises can be performed lying down, sitting, kneeling, or standing. By adjusting the tension and position, the Reformer provides endless variations for strengthening the core.

1. **Key Reformer Exercises for Core Strength:**
   - **Long Stretch:** This full-body exercise engages the core, shoulders, and legs by requiring you to maintain a plank-like position while the carriage moves.
   - **Knee Stretch:** Performed in a kneeling position, this exercise targets the lower abdominals and hip flexors as you move the carriage in and out using your core.
   - **Elephant:** In this standing exercise, you push the carriage with your legs while maintaining a strong core to stabilize your upper body.
2. **Core Benefits of Using the Reformer:**
   - The **Reformer** allows for dynamic movements that challenge the core in different planes of motion.
   - By providing resistance through springs, the **Reformer** increases the intensity of core exercises, helping to build strength and endurance.

- o The **Reformer** supports alignment and form, making it easier to perform complex movements with precision.

Summary

Advanced core Pilates exercises challenge your strength, coordination, and flexibility by incorporating full-body movements and precise control. Exercises like the **Teaser**, **Corkscrew**, and **Jackknife** require deep core engagement and build overall body awareness. Introducing the **Pilates Reformer** to your practice further enhances your core strength by adding resistance and variety. As you continue to progress, these advanced exercises will help you develop a stronger, more flexible, and resilient core, preparing you for even more challenging Pilates work.

Part 3: Flexibility-Focused Pilates Exercises

Chapter 7: Stretching and Strengthening for Flexibility

Flexibility is an integral component of overall fitness and well-being. In Pilates, flexibility complements strength by allowing your muscles to move through their full range of motion, which promotes fluidity, balance, and injury prevention. In this chapter, we explore stretching techniques that can help you achieve greater flexibility and strength in your Pilates practice, focusing on both **dynamic** and **static** stretches.

Dynamic vs. Static Stretching: Understanding the Two Types of Stretching

In Pilates, stretching is used both to increase range of motion and to prepare the body for movement. Understanding the difference between **dynamic** and **static** stretching is essential for optimizing your flexibility training.

Dynamic Stretching

Dynamic stretching involves moving your muscles and joints through a full range of motion in a controlled, continuous manner. These stretches are often used as part of a warm-up because they increase blood flow to the muscles and prepare them for more intense activity.

- **Examples in Pilates**:
    - **Leg Circles**: This classic Pilates exercise involves circling one leg in the air while lying on your back, which helps to open the hips and stretch the hamstrings dynamically.
    - **Arm Circles**: Standing or seated, extend your arms and make small circles to warm up the shoulder joints and muscles.

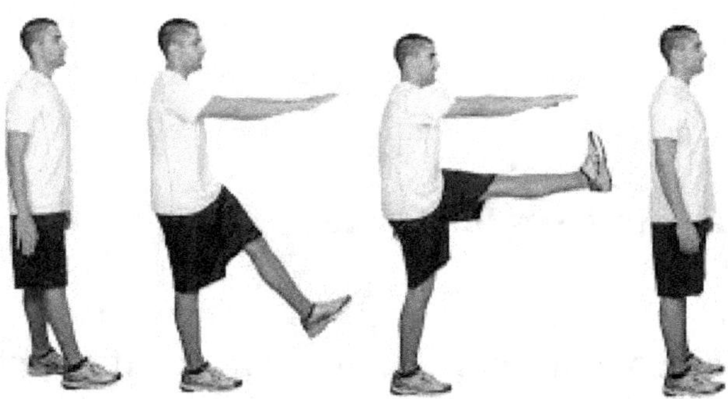

Static Stretching

Static stretching involves holding a stretch for an extended period, usually 15-60 seconds, to lengthen the muscles and increase flexibility. Static stretches are typically done after a workout to cool down or at the end of a flexibility-focused Pilates session.

- **Examples in Pilates**:
    - **Hamstring Stretch**: While lying on your back, extend one leg toward the ceiling, holding onto your ankle or calf, and feel the stretch in the back of your thigh.

- Spine Stretch Forward: Sitting tall with legs extended, reach forward toward your toes while rounding your back, which helps to stretch the spine and hamstrings.

Both types of stretching play a crucial role in Pilates. Dynamic stretches prepare the body for movement by warming up the muscles, while static stretches promote flexibility and relaxation at the end of a session.

Basic Stretches for Flexibility

While Pilates movements incorporate stretching throughout the practice, there are specific stretches that are particularly effective for increasing flexibility. Below are some basic stretches you can incorporate into your Pilates routine to target key areas of the body.

Hamstring Stretch

The **Hamstring Stretch** is one of the most fundamental stretches in Pilates and helps lengthen the muscles along the back of your thighs. Tight hamstrings can restrict movement and contribute to lower back pain, so this stretch is essential for improving overall mobility.

1. **How to Perform:**

o   Lie on your back with both legs extended.
o   Lift one leg toward the ceiling, keeping it straight while holding onto your ankle, calf, or thigh.
o   Flex your foot to deepen the stretch, and keep your other leg grounded on the mat.
o   Hold the stretch for 20-30 seconds, then switch legs.

2. **Tips for Deepening the Stretch:**
    o   If you have tight hamstrings, bend your knee slightly or use a strap to hold onto your leg.
    o   Focus on maintaining a neutral spine and avoid rounding your back.

3. **Benefits:**
    o   This stretch lengthens the hamstrings and calf muscles, improving flexibility in the legs and lower back. It also helps to release tension in the hips.

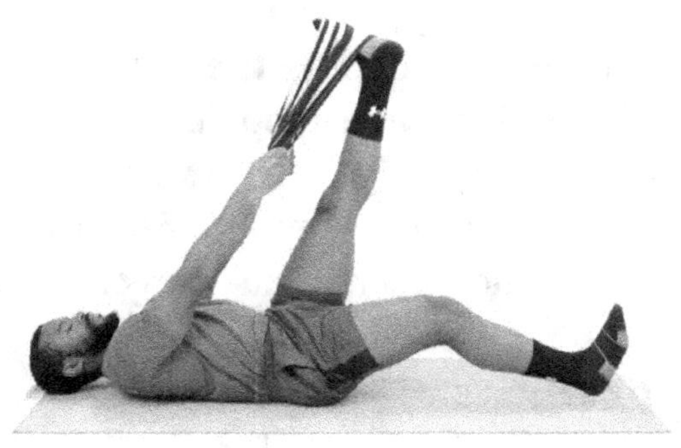

Spine Stretch Forward

The **Spine Stretch Forward** is a classic Pilates movement that lengthens the spine while stretching the hamstrings and back muscles. This stretch encourages mobility in the vertebrae and promotes good posture by targeting the muscles that support the spine.

1. **How to Perform:**
   - Sit tall on the mat with your legs extended straight in front of you, feet flexed, and arms extended forward.
   - Inhale as you lengthen through your spine, sitting as tall as possible.
   - Exhale as you slowly round your back, reaching your arms forward toward your toes.
   - Focus on articulating each vertebra as you fold forward, keeping your legs straight and feet flexed.
   - Hold for a few breaths, then inhale as you stack your spine back up to a tall sitting position.
2. **Tips for Deepening the Stretch:**
   - Keep your shoulders relaxed and avoid hunching them toward your ears.
   - Engage your core to support the movement and prevent collapsing into the stretch.
3. **Benefits:**
   - The **Spine Stretch Forward** increases flexibility in the hamstrings and lower back while promoting spinal mobility. It

also helps to relieve tension in the upper and middle back, making it a great stretch for those with sedentary lifestyles or poor posture.

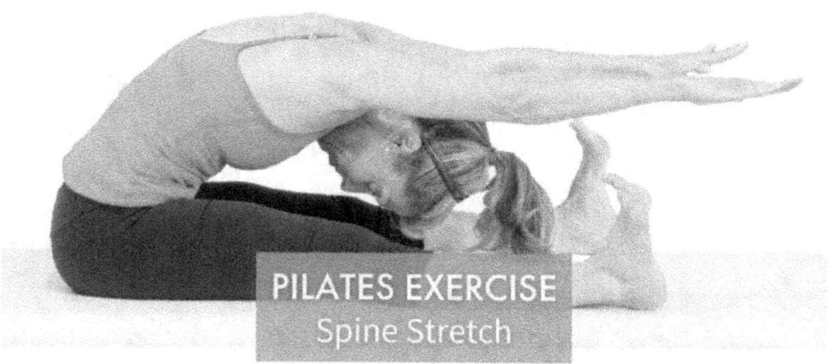

Shoulder Roll

The **Shoulder Roll** is a gentle yet effective stretch that helps release tension in the shoulders and upper back. This stretch can be performed at any point during your Pilates session and is particularly useful for improving flexibility in the shoulder girdle.

1. **How to Perform:**
   - Sit or stand tall with your arms by your sides.
   - Inhale as you lift your shoulders up toward your ears.
   - Exhale as you roll your shoulders back and down, opening your chest and

allowing your shoulder blades to slide together.

- o Repeat this movement 5-10 times, then reverse the direction by rolling your shoulders forward.

2. **Tips for Deepening the Stretch:**
   - o Focus on making the movement as smooth and controlled as possible.
   - o Keep your neck long and avoid tensing your jaw.

3. **Benefits:**
   - o The **Shoulder Roll** stretches the muscles in the shoulders and upper back, improving flexibility in the shoulder joints and releasing tightness caused by stress or poor posture. It's also an excellent way to improve shoulder mobility, which is important for many Pilates exercises.

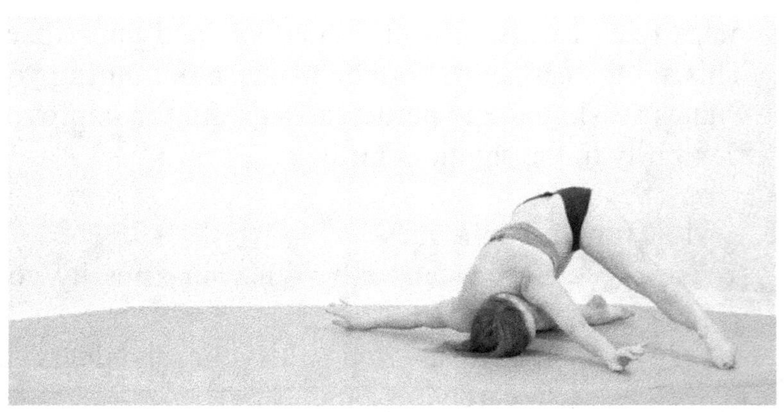

Summary

Flexibility is key to a well-rounded Pilates practice, enhancing movement quality and reducing the risk of injury. By understanding the difference between dynamic and static stretching, you can tailor your Pilates routine to improve flexibility in the key muscle groups such as the hamstrings, spine, and shoulders. Incorporating stretches like the **Hamstring Stretch**, **Spine Stretch Forward**, and **Shoulder Roll** into your Pilates sessions will help you build a more mobile and balanced body. As you progress in your flexibility journey, remember to listen to your body and use your breath to guide each stretch, ensuring a safe and effective practice.

Chapter 8: Flexibility through Pilates Flow

Flexibility is not only about stretching individual muscles but about integrating movement patterns that promote fluidity and balance throughout the entire body. Pilates incorporates a variety of exercises that not only enhance strength but also promote flexibility, allowing the body to move with greater ease and range. In this chapter, we'll explore some Pilates exercises specifically designed to improve flexibility and how you can create a balanced routine to support overall mobility and functional movement.

Pilates Moves That Enhance Flexibility

The following Pilates exercises are designed to stretch and lengthen key muscle groups while promoting overall flexibility in the body. These movements also help develop strength and coordination, offering a balanced approach to flexibility training.

Swan Dive

The **Swan Dive** is a dynamic Pilates exercise that focuses on back extension, helping to stretch and lengthen the spine and open the chest. This movement strengthens the muscles of the back while increasing flexibility in the spine, shoulders, and chest.

1. **How to Perform:**
    - Lie face down on your mat with your arms extended in front of you and your legs straight.
    - Engage your core and press your palms into the mat as you lift your chest off the ground, extending through your spine.
    - Keep your head in line with your spine, and lengthen your legs, allowing your upper body to arch backward.
    - Once you've reached your highest point, release your hands and rock forward, maintaining control through your core, and return to the starting position.
    - Repeat 5-8 times.
2. **Tips for Deepening the Stretch:**
    - Focus on lengthening through the crown of your head and reaching through your toes to maximize the stretch.
    - Avoid overarching your lower back by engaging your glutes and abdominals to support the movement.
3. **Benefits:**
    - The **Swan Dive** increases flexibility in the spine and chest while also strengthening the back extensors. It's a great exercise for counteracting poor posture caused by sitting and slouching.

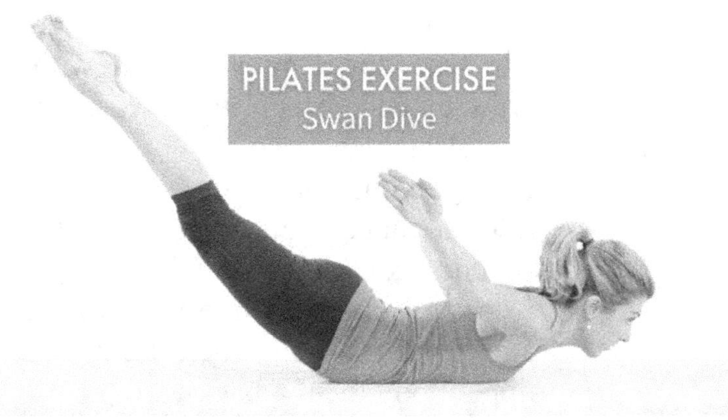

Single-Leg Circles

Single-Leg Circles are an effective exercise for increasing flexibility in the hips, hamstrings, and lower back. This movement also helps to improve coordination and balance while strengthening the core.

1. **How to Perform:**
   - Lie on your back with one leg extended toward the ceiling and the other leg flat on the mat.
   - Keep your arms by your sides and your core engaged.
   - Slowly circle the raised leg in one direction, making sure to keep your hips stable.
   - Complete 5-8 circles, then reverse the direction.
   - Switch legs and repeat on the other side.
2. **Tips for Deepening the Stretch:**

- o Keep your raised leg as straight as possible and your toes pointed to feel a deep stretch through your hamstrings.
  - o Focus on controlling the movement and keeping your pelvis stable, rather than letting your hips rotate with the leg.
3. **Benefits:**
  - o This exercise stretches the hamstrings and hip flexors, while also enhancing mobility in the hip joint. It's particularly effective for people with tight hips and lower back stiffness.

Mermaid Stretch

The **Mermaid Stretch** is a lateral stretch that focuses on increasing flexibility in the sides of the body, particularly the obliques, intercostal muscles, and lower back. It also helps to open the hips and chest, making it an excellent exercise for improving overall mobility.

1. **How to Perform:**
  - o Sit on your mat with your legs bent to the side, stacking your knees together, and placing your left hand on the floor beside you.
  - o Reach your right arm overhead, lengthening through your fingertips.

- o Inhale as you stretch your torso to the left, feeling the stretch along the right side of your body.
  - o Exhale as you return to an upright position.
  - o Repeat 5-8 times on each side.
2. **Tips for Deepening the Stretch:**
  - o Keep your shoulders relaxed and away from your ears to maximize the stretch through your sides.
  - o Imagine creating space between each rib as you stretch to promote length and flexibility.
3. **Benefits:**
  - o The **Mermaid Stretch** helps to lengthen the obliques and intercostal muscles, improving flexibility in the torso and enhancing side-bending movements. It's particularly beneficial for releasing tension in the lower back and hips.

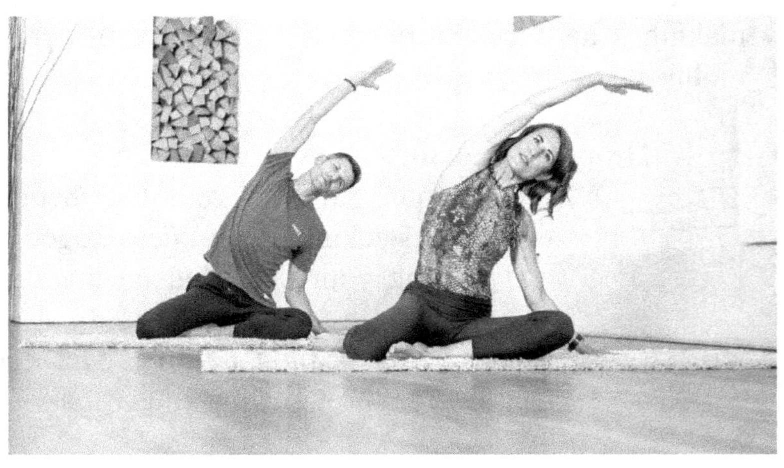

Creating Flexibility Routines

One of the key advantages of Pilates is its ability to combine flexibility and strength in a fluid, balanced routine. By incorporating a variety of flexibility-enhancing movements, you can develop a routine that not only stretches your muscles but also improves overall functional movement.

1. Balance Strength and Stretching

A well-rounded Pilates routine should include both flexibility and strength-based exercises. For instance, you can combine moves like the **Swan Dive**, which focuses on strength and extension, with the **Mermaid Stretch**, which promotes lateral flexibility. This combination helps to balance the body and prevent muscular imbalances.

2. Focus on Full-Body Movement

Flexibility routines should not only target specific muscle groups but should incorporate full-body movements that promote coordination and flow. Exercises like the **Single-Leg Circles** enhance flexibility in the hips and hamstrings while engaging the core, making them effective for improving mobility in multiple areas of the body at once.

3. Use Flow for Enhanced Flexibility

Pilates is known for its flowing movements, which means transitions between exercises should be smooth and controlled. By focusing on flow, you can enhance flexibility by keeping the body in motion, rather than performing isolated stretches. For example, transitioning from the **Single-Leg Circles** to the **Mermaid Stretch** helps to stretch both the lower and upper body in one continuous movement.

4. Progressive Stretching

Just like strength training, flexibility can be progressively improved over time. Start with basic stretches, such as hamstring or spine stretches, and gradually introduce more advanced moves like the **Swan Dive** or **Teaser**. This progressive approach ensures that you safely build flexibility while avoiding overstretching or injury.

Summary

Flexibility is a key component of Pilates that enhances not only mobility but also strength and functional movement. By incorporating Pilates exercises such as the **Swan Dive**, **Single-Leg Circles**, and **Mermaid Stretch**, you can develop a more flexible, balanced body. Creating a flow-based flexibility routine that integrates strength and mobility will allow you to move with greater ease and fluidity in everyday life. Remember to approach flexibility progressively, using both static and dynamic stretches to ensure safe and effective results.

Chapter 9: Advanced Flexibility Work in Pilates

As you progress in your Pilates journey, it's important to explore advanced techniques that deepen your flexibility and enhance your overall practice. This chapter focuses on advanced stretching techniques and the use of specialized Pilates equipment like the Reformer and Cadillac to aid in achieving greater flexibility. By incorporating these advanced movements into your routine, you'll experience not only improved flexibility but also increased strength, stability, and body awareness.

Deep Stretching Techniques

Advanced flexibility work in Pilates often involves deeper stretching techniques that target multiple muscle groups while promoting overall body alignment and balance. Here are some key exercises to consider:

Leg Pull

The **Leg Pull** is a challenging exercise that promotes flexibility in the hamstrings and hip flexors while engaging the core and stabilizing muscles. This exercise also helps to improve balance and coordination.

1. **How to Perform:**
   - Begin in a plank position with your hands under your shoulders and your body in a straight line from head to heels.
   - Inhale as you lift one leg towards the ceiling, keeping it straight and engaging your core.
   - Hold for a moment, then exhale as you lower the leg back down.
   - Alternate lifting each leg for 5-8 repetitions.

2. **Tips for Deepening the Stretch:**
   - Keep your hips square and avoid letting them sag as you lift your leg.
   - Focus on keeping your core engaged to maintain stability throughout the movement.

3. **Benefits:**
   - The **Leg Pull** not only stretches the hamstrings but also strengthens the core, shoulders, and glutes, making it an effective full-body exercise. This movement increases flexibility in the back of the legs and enhances overall body awareness.

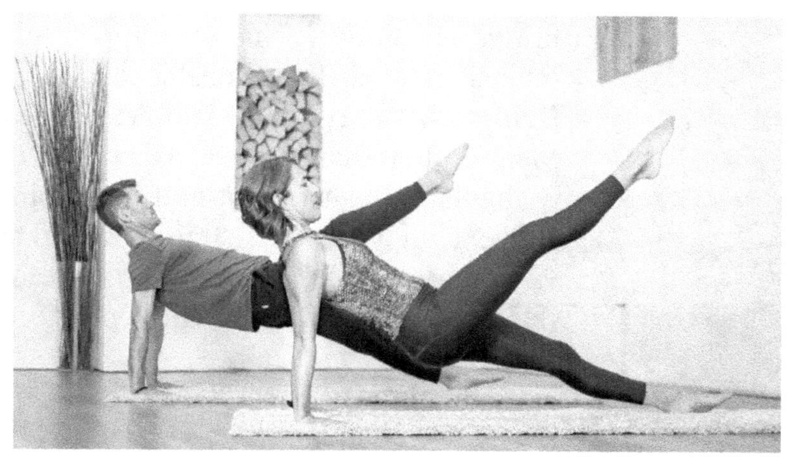

Bridge Variations

The **Bridge** is a versatile exercise that can be modified to increase flexibility and strengthen the posterior chain, including the glutes, hamstrings, and lower back. Advanced variations of the bridge can further enhance flexibility in the spine and hips.

1. **How to Perform the Basic Bridge:**
   - Lie on your back with your knees bent and feet flat on the mat, hip-width apart.
   - Press your feet into the ground and lift your hips towards the ceiling, engaging your glutes and core.
   - Hold the position for a few breaths, then slowly lower back down.
2. **Advanced Bridge Variations:**
   - **Single-Leg Bridge:** Lift one leg straight up toward the ceiling while holding the

bridge position. This variation adds intensity and challenges balance.

- o **Bridge with a Foam Roller:** Place a foam roller under your sacrum (the triangular bone at the base of your spine) and extend your legs straight out. This variation enhances the stretch in the hip flexors and spine while providing support.

3. **Tips for Deepening the Stretch:**
   - o Focus on engaging your core and squeezing your glutes as you lift to prevent arching your lower back.
   - o Experiment with arm positions, such as extending your arms overhead, to deepen the stretch in your shoulders and upper back.

4. **Benefits:**
   - o Bridge variations not only improve spinal flexibility but also strengthen the posterior chain, leading to better posture and reduced risk of injury. These movements enhance overall body awareness and control.

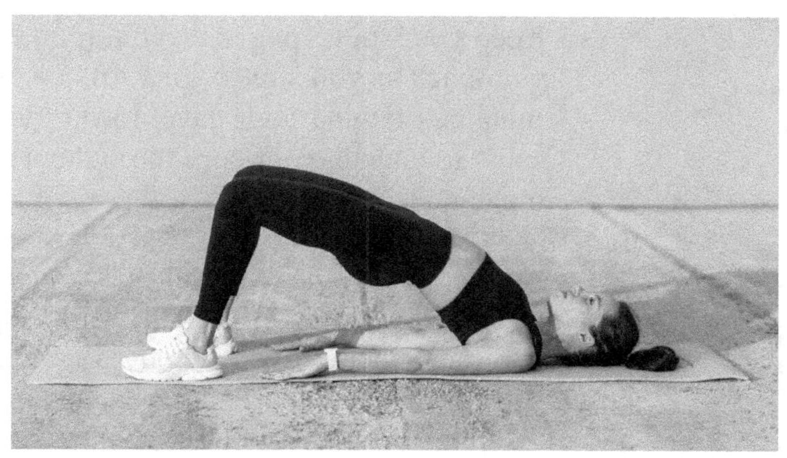

Advanced Spine Stretches

Advanced spine stretches target the flexibility of the spine and enhance the mobility of the thoracic and lumbar regions. These stretches help counteract the effects of prolonged sitting and improve overall posture.

1. **How to Perform an Advanced Spine Stretch:**
   - Sit up tall with your legs extended straight in front of you, feet flexed.
   - Inhale as you lengthen through your spine, reaching your arms overhead.
   - Exhale as you hinge forward from the hips, reaching toward your toes while maintaining a flat back.
   - Hold the stretch for a few breaths, then return to the starting position.
2. **Tips for Deepening the Stretch:**

- o Keep your spine long and avoid rounding your back as you stretch forward.
- o Imagine drawing your navel toward your spine to engage your core throughout the movement.

3. **Benefits:**
- o Advanced spine stretches promote flexibility in the back and hamstrings while enhancing overall body alignment and balance. These movements are essential for maintaining a healthy spine and preventing back pain.

Flexibility Training with Pilates Equipment

Incorporating Pilates equipment like the Reformer and Cadillac into your routine can significantly enhance your flexibility training. These pieces of equipment provide unique resistance and support, allowing for deeper stretches and improved alignment.

Using the Reformer for Flexibility

The Reformer is a versatile piece of equipment that allows for various exercises targeting flexibility, strength, and stability.

1. **Reformer Stretch Series:**

- Footwork Stretch: Place your feet on the footbar and press out while extending your legs. This movement provides resistance while stretching the calves and hamstrings.
  - **Kneeling Arm Reach:** Kneel on the carriage with one foot on the footbar. Reach the opposite arm overhead while extending your spine, allowing for a deep side stretch.
2. **Tips for Effective Use:**
   - Adjust the resistance on the Reformer to ensure you can maintain control while stretching.
   - Focus on slow, controlled movements to maximize the benefits of each stretch.
3. **Benefits:**
   - Using the Reformer allows for targeted stretching and strengthening of specific muscle groups while improving overall alignment and flexibility.

Using the Cadillac for Flexibility

The Cadillac, also known as the Trapeze Table, is an excellent tool for deepening stretches and enhancing flexibility.

1. **Cadillac Stretch Series:**
   - **Leg Springs Stretch:** Lie on your back with your feet in the straps. Extend your

legs while pulling the springs, allowing for a deep stretch in the hamstrings and lower back.

- o **Swan Stretch on Cadillac:** Position yourself on the Cadillac with your hands on the bars. As you extend your spine and lift your chest, feel the stretch along your back and shoulders.

2. **Tips for Effective Use:**
   - o Use the springs to provide gentle resistance while stretching, allowing for deeper movements.
   - o Maintain control and focus on alignment to prevent injury.

3. **Benefits:**
   - o The Cadillac enhances flexibility by providing support during stretches, allowing for more profound and controlled movements that target multiple muscle groups.

Summary

Advanced flexibility work in Pilates involves deep stretching techniques that target specific muscle groups and enhance overall mobility. Exercises such as the **Leg Pull**, **Bridge Variations**, and advanced spine stretches promote flexibility while improving strength and body awareness. Utilizing Pilates equipment like the Reformer and Cadillac allows for targeted stretching and deeper engagement, leading to improved alignment and functional movement. By integrating these advanced techniques into your Pilates practice, you can achieve a balanced and flexible body, enhancing your overall well-being and performance in daily activities.

Part 4: Integrating Core Strength and Flexibility in Pilates Workouts

Chapter 10: Pilates Routines for Core Strength and Flexibility

In this chapter, we will explore how to effectively combine core-focused and flexibility-focused exercises into balanced Pilates routines that not only enhance core strength and flexibility but also promote overall body awareness, alignment, and functional movement. Whether you are a beginner or an experienced practitioner, these routines will help you maximize the benefits of your Pilates practice and create a harmonious balance between strength and flexibility.

Balanced Routines

Creating a balanced routine in Pilates involves strategically combining core-strengthening and flexibility-enhancing exercises to promote overall wellness. A well-structured routine can improve your body's stability, enhance mobility, and reduce the risk of injury. Below are some key principles to consider when designing balanced Pilates routines:

1. **Integrating Core and Flexibility:**
   - **Focus on Transitioning:** Move seamlessly from core exercises to flexibility stretches to maintain a flow that keeps the body engaged. For

example, follow a core exercise with a gentle stretch to release tension in the muscles worked.

- o **Choose Complementary Exercises:** Pair exercises that work synergistically, such as combining a core-strengthening exercise like the **Plank** with a flexibility move like the **Cat-Cow Stretch**, which helps release tension in the back.

2. **Structuring Your Routine:**

- o **Warm-Up:** Begin with a brief warm-up that activates the core and prepares the body for movement. Incorporate exercises like **Pelvic Tilts** or **Arm Circles** to increase blood flow and mobility.
- o **Core Strengthening Segment:** Include exercises that specifically target core strength, such as the **Hundred, Roll-Up,** or **Double Leg Stretch**.
- o **Flexibility Segment:** Follow the core exercises with stretches that promote flexibility, such as the **Spine Stretch Forward** and **Hamstring Stretch**.
- o **Cool Down:** End with a cool-down that includes deep breathing and gentle stretches, such as the **Child's Pose** or **Seated Forward Bend**, to relax and restore the body.

Full-Body Workouts

To make the most of your Pilates practice, we'll provide a full-body workout routine that combines core-strengthening and flexibility exercises into a cohesive 30-minute session. This routine can be performed on a mat or with the aid of Pilates equipment, depending on your experience level and available resources.

30-Minute Full-Body Pilates Routine

Warm-Up (5 minutes):

- **Pelvic Tilts (1 minute):** Lie on your back with knees bent and feet flat. Inhale to prepare, then exhale as you gently tilt your pelvis, flattening your lower back against the mat. Inhale to release.
- **Arm Circles (1 minute):** Stand or sit with your arms extended to the sides. Make small circles forward for 30 seconds, then reverse for another 30 seconds.

Core Strengthening Segment (15 minutes):

1. **The Hundred (2 minutes):**
    - Lie on your back, lift your legs to a tabletop position, and curl your head and shoulders off the mat. Pump your arms up and down while breathing in for five counts and out for five counts until you reach 100.
2. **Roll-Up (2 minutes):**

- Lie flat with arms overhead. Inhale to prepare, then exhale as you roll up one vertebra at a time, reaching toward your toes. Inhale as you roll back down.

3. **Double Leg Stretch (2 minutes):**
   - From a supine position, pull your knees to your chest. Inhale as you extend your arms and legs out, exhale to return to the starting position.

4. **Plank (2 minutes):**
   - From a push-up position, engage your core and hold for 30 seconds. Rest briefly and repeat for another 30 seconds.

5. **Side Plank (2 minutes):**
   - Lie on your side with legs stacked. Prop yourself on your elbow and lift your hips off the mat. Hold for 30 seconds on each side.

6. **Criss-Cross (2 minutes):**
   - Lie on your back with knees bent. Lift your head and shoulders, and bring one elbow toward the opposite knee while extending the other leg. Alternate sides for one minute.

7. **Bridge (2 minutes):**
   - Lie on your back with knees bent and feet hip-width apart. Press through your feet to lift your hips, engaging your glutes and hamstrings. Hold for a few seconds and lower down.

Flexibility Segment (10 minutes):

1. **Spine Stretch Forward (2 minutes):**
   - o Sit tall with legs extended. Inhale to lengthen, exhale as you reach forward toward your toes, feeling the stretch in your hamstrings and spine.
2. **Hamstring Stretch (2 minutes):**
   - o From a seated position, extend one leg out and bend the other. Reach towards the extended foot, feeling the stretch in the hamstring. Hold for 30 seconds on each leg.
3. **Cat-Cow Stretch (2 minutes):**
   - o Start on all fours. Inhale as you arch your back and look up (cow position), then exhale as you round your spine (cat position). Repeat for one minute.
4. **Seated Forward Bend (2 minutes):**
   - o Sit with legs extended. Inhale to prepare, exhale as you hinge at the hips and reach toward your feet, feeling the stretch along the spine and hamstrings.
5. **Child's Pose (2 minutes):**
   - o Kneel on the mat and sit back on your heels. Reach your arms forward and relax your forehead on the mat. Breathe deeply to release tension.

Cool Down (5 minutes):

- **Breath Awareness (2 minutes):** Sit cross-legged or lie flat. Focus on your breath, inhaling deeply through the nose and exhaling slowly through the mouth.

- **Gentle Neck Rolls (1 minute):** Gently roll your head side to side and forward, releasing any remaining tension.
- **Final Stretch (2 minutes):** Extend your arms overhead and stretch your whole body, then relax.

Conclusion

This chapter provided you with a comprehensive approach to creating balanced Pilates routines that integrate core-strengthening and flexibility-enhancing exercises. By focusing on the principles of Pilates and incorporating targeted movements, you can develop a well-rounded practice that supports your overall health and wellness. With consistency and dedication, these routines will help you build a strong core, increase flexibility, and foster a deeper connection between your mind and body. Enjoy the journey of transformation that Pilates offers!

Chapter 11: Customizing Your Pilates Practice

In this chapter, we will explore how to tailor your Pilates practice to meet your individual needs, fitness levels, and personal goals. Pilates is a versatile method that can be adjusted to suit a wide range of abilities and objectives. Whether you're a beginner, an intermediate practitioner, or advanced, customizing your practice can lead to more effective workouts and a greater sense of accomplishment.

Tailoring Pilates to Your Needs

One of the fundamental strengths of Pilates is its adaptability. Below are strategies on how to customize your Pilates practice based on different factors:

1. **Assessing Your Fitness Level:**
   - **Beginner:** If you're new to Pilates, start with foundational exercises that focus on core engagement, alignment, and breathing. Simple movements like the **Pelvic Tilt** and **Arm Circles** help establish a strong base.
   - **Intermediate:** Once you're comfortable with the basics, progress to intermediate exercises that introduce more complexity, such as the **Roll-Up** and **Plank Variations**. These exercises build on your existing strength and flexibility.

- **Advanced:** Advanced practitioners can explore challenging movements like the **Teaser** and **Jackknife**, as well as using Pilates equipment like the Reformer for enhanced resistance and support.

2. **Adapting Exercises for Flexibility:**
   - **Limited Flexibility:** If you struggle with flexibility, focus on gentler stretches and modifications. Utilize props such as resistance bands or blocks to assist in poses like the **Hamstring Stretch**.
   - **Improving Flexibility:** Incorporate dynamic stretching techniques, such as the **Swan Dive** and **Mermaid Stretch**, to gently push your limits without risking injury.

3. **Incorporating Modifications:**
   - **Use of Props:** Props like a Pilates ring, stability ball, or foam roller can help modify exercises to suit your needs. For example, placing a ball under your lower back during the **Bridge** can provide additional support.
   - **Body Positioning:** Adjusting your positioning can make exercises more accessible. If a movement feels too challenging, try performing it on your knees instead of your toes, or with one leg grounded for balance.

4. **Listening to Your Body:**
   - Pay attention to how your body feels during each exercise. If something feels uncomfortable or painful, modify or skip

that movement. This self-awareness is key to a safe and effective Pilates practice.

Setting Goals for Core Strength and Flexibility

Establishing clear, achievable goals is essential for maintaining motivation and tracking progress. Here are strategies to help you set and personalize your goals:

1. **SMART Goals:**
   - **Specific:** Define your goals clearly. Instead of saying, "I want to be more flexible," specify, "I want to be able to touch my toes in three months."
   - **Measurable:** Set measurable criteria to track your progress. For example, aim to increase your **Hamstring Stretch** by a certain number of inches over a set timeframe.
   - **Achievable:** Ensure your goals are realistic and attainable, considering your current fitness level and lifestyle.
   - **Relevant:** Your goals should align with your overall health and fitness aspirations. If improving core strength is your focus, prioritize exercises that target this area.
   - **Time-bound:** Set deadlines for your goals to create urgency and commitment. For instance, "I want to complete a 30-

minute Pilates session three times a week for the next month."

2. **Tracking Progress:**
    - **Journaling:** Keep a Pilates journal where you can note down your routines, exercises performed, and any changes in flexibility or strength. This documentation can help you see your growth over time.
    - **Photos and Measurements:** Take photos or measurements of your progress. For instance, measure your flexibility using a measuring tape to track how far you can reach during stretches.

3. **Adjusting Goals as Needed:**
    - As you progress, be open to adjusting your goals. If you find that a specific target has been met, set new ones that challenge you further.
    - Don't hesitate to modify your goals based on changes in your lifestyle or fitness levels. Flexibility is key in a successful Pilates journey.

4. **Creating a Balanced Routine:**
    - **Core and Flexibility Balance:** Design a routine that incorporates both core-strengthening and flexibility-enhancing exercises. For example, alternate between core exercises like **The Hundred** and stretches like the **Spine Stretch Forward** within your weekly workouts.

- o **Weekly Schedule:** Establish a weekly schedule that includes specific days for core-focused workouts and other days dedicated to flexibility training. This structure will help you achieve a harmonious balance.
5. **Involving a Professional:**
   - o If possible, consider working with a certified Pilates instructor who can help personalize your practice based on your individual needs. An instructor can provide valuable feedback, introduce new exercises, and ensure you're performing movements safely and effectively.

Customizing your Pilates practice allows you to harness the full potential of this mind-body discipline. By tailoring exercises to suit your fitness level, personal goals, and individual needs, you create a practice that is not only enjoyable but also effective. Setting clear goals and regularly assessing your progress will keep you motivated and moving forward on your journey toward enhanced core strength and flexibility. Remember, Pilates is a lifelong practice, and every step you take brings you closer to your ideal self. Enjoy the process, celebrate your achievements, and continue to evolve your practice for a healthier, more balanced life!

Part 5: Long-Term Strategies for Pilates Success

Chapter 12: Building a Sustainable Pilates Routine

Establishing a sustainable Pilates routine is key to experiencing the long-term benefits of strength, flexibility, and mindfulness. In this chapter, we'll explore how to stay consistent, track your progress, and modify your practice as you become stronger and more flexible.

Staying Consistent: How to Maintain Regular Practice and Keep Progressing

Consistency is the cornerstone of any successful fitness journey. When it comes to Pilates, regular practice ensures that the improvements in core strength, flexibility, and overall well-being continue to build over time. To maintain consistency, consider the following strategies:

1. **Set a Realistic Schedule**
   Aiming for daily practice might be overwhelming for beginners, so it's important to start with a realistic and achievable routine. Start by committing to 3–4 Pilates sessions per week, gradually increasing the frequency as your endurance and enthusiasm grow. Choose times that fit seamlessly into your daily schedule, whether it's a morning routine to energize your day or an evening wind-down session to relax your mind and body.

2. **Create a Dedicated Practice Space**
Having a designated space for your Pilates practice can help signal your brain that it's time to exercise. Whether it's a corner of your living room or a private room in your home, ensure the space is free of distractions and clutter. Equip it with the basics like a yoga mat, resistance bands, or Pilates ball. A calming environment, perhaps with soft lighting or soothing music, can make your practice something to look forward to.

3. **Set Small, Achievable Goals**
Rather than focusing on distant goals like perfecting a challenging move, break them down into smaller, actionable steps. For instance, aim to hold a plank for an extra five seconds or increase the depth of your stretches each week. Small wins help build momentum and keep you motivated as you see progress over time.

4. **Mix It Up**
Doing the same routine repeatedly can lead to boredom or plateaus. To stay engaged, incorporate variety into your workouts by alternating between different types of Pilates exercises. This could include focusing on different muscle groups, incorporating equipment like resistance bands or Pilates balls, or alternating between mat Pilates and reformer-based exercises if available.

5. **Find Accountability**
Consistency is easier when you have support. Consider joining a class, either in person or

online, where you can find encouragement and motivation from instructors and fellow practitioners. If classes aren't feasible, try practicing with a friend or partner. Having an accountability partner can provide extra motivation, and the shared experience may help deepen your commitment to Pilates.

6. **Listen to Your Body**
   Consistency doesn't mean pushing through pain or fatigue. Rest is an essential component of any sustainable fitness routine. If you're feeling sore or overworked, allow yourself to take a day off or engage in a restorative Pilates session with a focus on gentle movements and deep stretching. By respecting your body's signals, you'll maintain long-term sustainability.

Measuring Your Progress: How to Track Improvements in Core Strength and Flexibility Over Time

Tracking your progress is essential for staying motivated and identifying areas for improvement. Pilates is unique in that the benefits aren't always immediately visible, but with patience and dedication, you'll notice significant changes in how your body feels and moves. Here are a few ways to measure your progress effectively:

1. **Keep a Pilates Journal**
   Documenting your practice is a great way to track your physical and mental progress. Record the exercises you performed, the duration of

your practice, and any challenges you encountered. Over time, this log will provide a clear picture of how far you've come, whether it's increased flexibility, longer plank holds, or improved posture.

2. **Set Benchmarks for Strength and Flexibility** Establish baseline measurements of your core strength and flexibility when you begin your Pilates journey. For strength, you could measure how long you can hold a plank or perform controlled push-ups. For flexibility, note how far you can reach in a seated forward bend or the depth of your squats. Reassess these benchmarks every month or so to track your progress.

3. **Take Progress Photos or Videos** Pilates often creates subtle physical changes in the body, such as improved posture, lean muscle tone, and enhanced flexibility. Taking progress photos or videos at regular intervals can help you visualize these improvements. Before-and-after photos of your posture, for instance, can reveal how Pilates has helped align your spine or open your shoulders.

4. **Pay Attention to Daily Activities** One of the great benefits of Pilates is its positive impact on everyday movements. Notice how your body feels during activities like carrying groceries, walking up stairs, or even sitting at a desk. As your core becomes stronger and your flexibility improves, you should find these tasks easier and less fatiguing. Recognizing how Pilates supports your

functional strength is another way to measure progress.

5. **Mental and Emotional Growth**
   Pilates is as much a mental practice as it is a physical one. As you continue, you may notice an increased sense of mental clarity, reduced stress, or enhanced mindfulness. These mental benefits are often just as important as the physical changes and contribute to a well-rounded Pilates experience.

Modifying Your Practice as You Improve: Adjusting Your Routine as You Grow Stronger and More Flexible

As you progress in your Pilates journey, it's crucial to adapt your routine to match your growing strength and flexibility. Sticking to the same beginner exercises might hinder your growth, so gradually advancing your practice will ensure continued improvement.

1. **Increase the Intensity**
   Once you've mastered the basics, start adding more challenging exercises or variations to your routine. For example, you can modify the classic plank by transitioning to side planks or adding leg lifts to make it more difficult. You might also explore intermediate moves like the "Teaser" or "Side Leg Series," which require more control and balance.

2. **Add Resistance or Props**
   Incorporating resistance into your Pilates practice is another effective way to increase the

difficulty. Using resistance bands, small weights, or a Pilates ring can add an extra layer of challenge to your exercises. For instance, you can use a resistance band around your thighs during squats or leg lifts to engage your muscles more deeply.

3. **Lengthen or Intensify Your Sessions** As your endurance grows, consider extending the duration of your Pilates sessions or increasing the intensity of your exercises. If you initially practiced for 20–30 minutes, gradually build up to 45–60 minutes. Alternatively, you could perform more sets or reduce rest periods between exercises for a more intense workout.

4. **Focus on Advanced Movements** Once you've gained confidence in your form and core strength, begin incorporating advanced Pilates movements. Exercises like the "Swan Dive," "Roll Over," or "Scissors" challenge the body in new ways, promoting further flexibility, coordination, and muscle control.

5. **Listen to Your Changing Body** As you progress, you might find that certain areas of your body need more attention. For example, if your core strength has improved, but your hamstrings feel tight, you can adjust your routine to focus more on stretching and lengthening those muscles. Likewise, if you feel tension in your neck or lower back, modify your exercises to prevent strain and discomfort.

6. **Explore Different Pilates Modalities** Expanding your Pilates repertoire can also include exploring different forms of the

practice, such as reformer Pilates, Pilates with a stability ball, or combining Pilates with other fitness modalities like yoga or barre. These variations will keep your routine fresh, engage different muscle groups, and provide new challenges.

Building a sustainable Pilates routine is a long-term commitment that rewards you with not only physical strength and flexibility but also mental clarity and emotional resilience. With consistency, proper tracking, and routine modifications, you'll continue to experience growth and progress in your Pilates practice, creating a strong foundation for lifelong fitness and well-being.

Chapter 13: Incorporating Pilates into Your Daily Life

Pilates is not just about dedicated workouts; it can become a part of your daily routine, enhancing your posture, core strength, flexibility, and overall mobility throughout the day. This chapter will explore how to seamlessly integrate Pilates into your everyday life, allowing you to experience its benefits even outside of your workout sessions.

Functional Core Strength: Using Pilates Exercises Throughout the Day to Support Posture, Stability, and Mobility

A strong core is at the heart of Pilates practice, and the benefits of functional core strength extend far beyond your mat or reformer. By incorporating core-focused movements throughout your day, you can support better posture, reduce back pain, and improve stability in everyday activities. Here's how:

1. **Posture Awareness at Work**
   Many people spend hours sitting at a desk, which can lead to slouching and poor posture. Pilates teaches awareness of body alignment and core engagement, which can be applied while sitting or standing. Throughout the day, remind yourself to sit tall, engage your core, and align your shoulders over your hips. You can even perform small, seated core activations, such as pelvic tilts or gentle seated twists, to

keep your muscles engaged during long periods of sitting.

2. **Core Engagement While Walking**
Walking is a great opportunity to apply Pilates principles. Focus on maintaining good posture by keeping your spine tall, your shoulders back, and your core lightly engaged. This alignment improves your gait, reduces strain on your lower back, and allows your core to support your movement. With regular practice, this awareness becomes second nature, turning walking into a functional core workout.

3. **Lifting and Carrying Objects**
Whether you're carrying groceries, lifting a heavy box, or picking up your child, Pilates principles can help you move safely and efficiently. Rather than relying on your lower back or shoulders to lift, engage your core and use your legs to power the movement. This helps prevent injury and strengthens your deep abdominal muscles. You can practice squats or lunges as a form of functional movement training to reinforce these healthy lifting habits.

4. **Balance and Stability Throughout the Day**
Balance is another key benefit of Pilates, and it can be cultivated in everyday activities. For example, while brushing your teeth, try standing on one leg for an extra balance challenge. This simple activity engages your core and stabilizing muscles, helping to improve balance and coordination. As your balance improves, you'll notice greater stability and control in other areas of your life, from

navigating uneven terrain to staying steady during sports or physical activities.

5. **Breathwork for Mindfulness and Core Engagement**

   Pilates emphasizes the connection between breath and movement. By practicing Pilates-style diaphragmatic breathing throughout the day, you can improve your oxygen intake, reduce stress, and keep your core muscles engaged. Take a few moments to practice deep belly breaths, expanding your ribcage as you inhale and contracting your abs as you exhale. This mindful breathing technique can help you stay calm and centered, while also activating your deep core muscles.

Pilates for Everyday Flexibility: How to Integrate Stretching Routines into Daily Activities for Continuous Flexibility Improvement

One of the major benefits of Pilates is the improvement in flexibility and mobility. Incorporating simple Pilates-inspired stretches into your daily life can help keep your muscles lengthened, reduce stiffness, and improve your overall range of motion.

1. **Morning Stretch Routine**

   Start your day with a few gentle Pilates stretches to wake up your body and prepare for the day ahead. Simple movements like spinal rolls, seated forward bends, and cat-cow stretches help mobilize the spine and warm up the muscles. These exercises can be done as soon as you wake up to loosen up tight muscles from sleep and set a positive tone for the rest of the day.

2. **Desk-Friendly Stretching**
   Long hours of sitting can cause tightness in the hips, shoulders, and back. To counteract this, incorporate brief stretching breaks into your workday. A seated spinal twist can release tension in your back, while a seated forward bend stretches the hamstrings and lower back. If possible, stand up periodically to perform hip stretches or shoulder rolls. These small movements help prevent stiffness and keep your muscles flexible throughout the day.

3. **Stretching While Watching TV**
   Leisure time doesn't have to be inactive. While watching TV, you can easily integrate stretches to improve your flexibility. Try lying on the floor in a supine position and gently stretching your hamstrings with a resistance band, or practice a spinal twist to release your back. Even a few minutes of stretching during a commercial break can enhance flexibility and reduce tension in your muscles.

4. **Pre- and Post-Workout Stretching**
   If you engage in other physical activities like running, cycling, or weightlifting, it's important to incorporate Pilates-based stretches to prevent injury and improve performance. Pre-workout stretches like leg swings and arm circles help to loosen up your muscles and prepare them for activity. Post-workout, static stretches such as hip flexor stretches, hamstring stretches, and

child's pose can aid in muscle recovery, reduce soreness, and promote flexibility.

5. **Evening Wind-Down Routine**
   Before going to bed, a short stretching routine can help you relax and unwind from the day's stresses. Focus on gentle stretches that target the muscles used most during the day, such as your lower back, hips, and shoulders. A few minutes of deep stretching paired with deep breathing can calm your mind, relieve tension, and promote better sleep.

6. **Integrating Dynamic Flexibility Movements**
   In addition to static stretches, Pilates incorporates dynamic flexibility exercises that combine movement with stretching. These can be integrated into your daily routine to improve mobility and flexibility over time. For example, movements like "leg circles" or "spine twists" not only stretch your muscles but also improve joint mobility and coordination. These exercises can be done during a warm-up or as part of a morning routine to increase flexibility and body awareness.

By incorporating Pilates exercises and stretches into your daily life, you'll enhance your core strength, posture, balance, and flexibility continuously. These small but powerful practices turn everyday moments into opportunities to engage your muscles and improve your overall well-being. With regular application, Pilates becomes more than just a workout—it becomes a way of moving and living with greater strength, mobility, and mindfulness.

Conclusion: The Journey to a Stronger, More Flexible You

As you reach the conclusion of this Pilates journey, it's important to take a moment to reflect on how far you've come and the transformation that's occurred, both physically and mentally. The practice of Pilates is more than just a fitness routine; it's a lifestyle that brings strength, flexibility, and a deeper connection to your body and mind.

Celebrating Progress: Reflecting on How Pilates Has Transformed Your Body and Mindset

Over the course of your Pilates practice, you've likely noticed significant changes in your body. Perhaps your core has become stronger, your posture has improved, and you feel more flexible and agile. But beyond the physical, Pilates often fosters a positive shift in mindset. Many practitioners report greater body awareness, reduced stress, and an improved sense of mental clarity.

Celebrating these milestones—whether they are in the form of increased strength, better flexibility, or more mindful movement—helps keep you motivated. Recognize the small victories, such as mastering a new exercise, improving your balance, or feeling more confident in your body. Reflecting on your progress will remind you that Pilates is not just about the destination but about enjoying the process of growth and self-improvement.

Continuing the Practice: Encouraging Long-Term Commitment to Pilates for Sustained Strength, Flexibility, and Overall Well-Being

Pilates is a lifelong practice, offering continuous benefits as you grow and evolve. While the exercises themselves help build and maintain muscle strength, improve flexibility, and promote core stability, the commitment to the practice also enhances your overall well-being. Regular Pilates sessions can prevent injury, support long-term mobility, and offer a much-needed break from the stresses of daily life.

To sustain these benefits, consistency is key. Whether it's carving out 10 minutes each morning for a few core exercises or dedicating time to a full routine a few times a week, staying committed to the practice will ensure that your hard-earned strength and flexibility remain with you. It's also helpful to stay engaged by mixing up your routines, challenging yourself with new exercises, and exploring different Pilates variations such as mat work, Reformer, or Pilates with props like resistance bands or stability balls.

Next Steps: How to Continue Advancing in Your Pilates Journey

As your journey continues, you may feel ready to take your practice to the next level. Pilates is a practice that allows for endless growth, and there are several avenues you can explore to keep things exciting and challenging:

1. **Reformer Work**
   The Pilates Reformer offers a dynamic way to advance your practice. This piece of equipment allows for a wider range of exercises and resistance training, providing new challenges for building strength, coordination, and flexibility. Reformer classes or personal sessions with a certified Pilates instructor can help you refine your technique and explore more advanced movements.

2. **Advanced Classes**
   As you become more confident in your abilities, consider enrolling in advanced Pilates classes. These classes often incorporate more complex sequences, faster transitions, and challenging exercises like teasers, rollovers, and advanced plank variations. Pushing yourself in these classes can deepen your practice and enhance your overall physical fitness.

3. **Pilates Teacher Training**
   If you've developed a passion for Pilates, you may even want to consider becoming a certified Pilates instructor. Teaching Pilates not only allows you to share the benefits with others but also reinforces your own understanding of the exercises and deepens your connection to the practice. Many Pilates teacher training programs offer comprehensive education on anatomy, biomechanics, and teaching techniques, setting you up for a rewarding career or a fulfilling hobby.

4. **Specialized Pilates Practices**
   Pilates offers a range of specialized programs,

from prenatal Pilates to Pilates for rehabilitation. Exploring these options can help you adapt your practice to different stages of life or specific needs. If you're recovering from an injury or going through a major life change, these targeted programs can provide tailored support and guidance.

5. **Cross-Training with Other Disciplines** You might also find it beneficial to complement your Pilates practice with other forms of exercise, such as yoga, strength training, or cardio. Each discipline offers unique benefits that can enhance your Pilates practice. For example, yoga improves flexibility and mental focus, strength training helps build muscle, and cardio supports cardiovascular health.

Final Thoughts

Your Pilates journey is not a linear path but rather a continuous cycle of learning, growing, and discovering new possibilities. Each step of the way, Pilates supports your strength, flexibility, and overall well-being, empowering you to move through life with greater ease and confidence. Keep celebrating your progress, stay consistent, and remain open to new challenges as you continue your journey to a stronger, more flexible you.

Appendices

Appendix A: Glossary of Pilates Terms

This section offers clear definitions of the key Pilates terms used throughout the book to ensure that practitioners of all levels can fully understand and implement the exercises.

- **Breath Control**: A fundamental principle of Pilates, focusing on deep and controlled breathing to engage the core and enhance movement.
- **Core**: Refers to the muscles of the abdomen, lower back, and pelvis, which are emphasized in Pilates for stability and strength.
- **Neutral Spine**: The position in which the natural curves of the spine are maintained during exercises to prevent injury and optimize alignment.
- **Flow**: Refers to the smooth, graceful, and continuous transition between Pilates movements.
- **Precision**: The emphasis on performing each exercise with proper form, alignment, and control.
- **Reformer**: A Pilates apparatus with a sliding carriage and adjustable springs, used to provide resistance for more dynamic and intense workouts.
- **Hundred**: A classic Pilates exercise involving core stability and strength, performed by

pumping the arms while holding a static "tabletop" or leg-extended position.

This glossary provides explanations of technical terminology, ensuring readers can easily follow the instructions and cues provided in the workout routines.

Appendix B: Suggested Pilates Equipment

While many Pilates exercises can be performed with just a mat, adding equipment and props can help enhance your practice by increasing resistance, improving balance, or adding variety. This guide will help you determine which tools are essential for your Pilates routine.

- **Yoga/Pilates Mat**: A thick, non-slip mat is essential for cushioning and comfort during floor exercises.
- **Resistance Bands**: Lightweight and versatile, these bands can be used to add resistance to various exercises, helping to build strength and flexibility.
- **Foam Roller**: An excellent tool for self-massage, improving mobility, and enhancing stretches. Foam rollers are also useful for balance and core stability exercises.
- **Pilates Ring (Magic Circle)**: A flexible ring that provides resistance during arm, leg, and core exercises. It's a simple yet effective tool for enhancing muscle engagement and increasing intensity.

- **Small Stability Ball**: A soft, inflatable ball used for core exercises and balance training, adding instability to the workout and increasing the challenge.
- **Reformer Machine**: Though not essential for beginners, the Reformer is a staple in Pilates studios. It uses springs and a sliding platform to intensify Pilates exercises, improving strength, flexibility, and coordination.
- **Ankle and Wrist Weights**: Light weights can be added to increase resistance and intensity in mat exercises.
- **Pilates Chair**: A compact apparatus used for seated or standing exercises that challenge balance and core strength while providing resistance with spring-loaded pedals.

By incorporating these tools into your practice, you can adapt your workouts to your fitness level and goals, allowing for continued progress and variety.

Appendix C: Sample Weekly Pilates Schedule

This appendix provides a pre-designed weekly schedule to help practitioners of all levels create a consistent and balanced Pilates practice. Each schedule can be adapted to suit your individual fitness goals and time constraints.

For Beginners:

- **Day 1**: Full-body mat routine (focus on core activation and basic exercises like the Hundred, leg lifts, and bridges)

- **Day 2**: Rest or gentle stretching
- **Day 3**: Lower body-focused routine (squats, lunges, and leg lifts with modifications)
- **Day 4**: Upper body and core (push-ups, planks, seated arm exercises with resistance bands)
- **Day 5**: Rest or light walk/stretch
- **Day 6**: Total body workout (mix of upper body, lower body, and core with Pilates ring and small stability ball)
- **Day 7**: Rest or gentle yoga

For Intermediate Practitioners:

- **Day 1**: Full-body workout using resistance bands and small weights (include planks, leg circles, and oblique twists)
- **Day 2**: Core and flexibility routine (target obliques and lower abs with exercises like side planks and Russian twists)
- **Day 3**: Rest day or mobility work (focus on stretching and foam rolling)
- **Day 4**: Lower body strength (Pilates ring exercises for glutes and thighs, squats with a small stability ball)
- **Day 5**: Upper body and core (use the Pilates ring and resistance bands for arm and core work)
- **Day 6**: Full-body Reformer session (if available) or more advanced mat routine (teasers, roll-ups, and Pilates push-ups)
- **Day 7**: Rest day or restorative stretching

For Advanced Practitioners:

- **Day 1**: Full-body Reformer workout (advanced exercises such as footwork, lunges, and coordination drills)
- **Day 2**: Upper body and core mat workout (focus on advanced moves like teaser, pike, and dynamic plank variations)
- **Day 3**: Rest or light flexibility work (emphasize mobility and recovery)
- **Day 4**: Lower body strength and mobility (challenging leg lifts, squats with resistance bands, and side-lying exercises)
- **Day 5**: Advanced core work (side planks, double leg stretch, and oblique exercises with weights)
- **Day 6**: Full-body Reformer or advanced mat Pilates with props (Pilates chair or resistance bands)
- **Day 7**: Rest or gentle movement (yoga, walking, or swimming)

These schedules can be used as a foundation for your weekly practice, helping you stay on track while ensuring you're targeting different muscle groups throughout the week. You can modify them as needed based on time availability and fitness level, ensuring long-term success in your Pilates journey.

www.ingramcontent.com/pod-product-compliance
Lightning Source LLC
Chambersburg PA
CBHW071043250726
48653CB00005B/1969